_f_**P**

THE
DETOX
—Vibrant Health In 5 Easy Steps—
STRATEGY

Brenda Watson, C.N.C.,
with Leonard Smith, M.D.

Free Press
New York London Toronto Sydney

Free Press
A Division of Simon & Schuster, Inc.
1230 Avenue of the Americas
New York, NY 10020

Copyright © 2008 by Brenda Watson
All rights reserved, including the right to reproduce
this book or portions thereof in any form whatsoever. For information address Free Press
Subsidiary Rights Department, 1230 Avenue of the Americas, New York, NY 10020

First Free Press trade paperback edition February 2009

FREE PRESS and colophon are trademarks of Simon & Schuster, Inc.

For information about special discounts for bulk purchases, please contact Simon & Schuster
Special Sales at 1-800-456-6798 or business@simonandschuster.com

Art Direction and Styling: michael black / BLACK SUN®
Graphic Design: Jason Oakman
Illustration: Nip Rogers

Manufactured in the United States of America

1   3   5   7   9   10   8   6   4   2

The Library of Congress has cataloged the hardcover edition as follows:
Watson, Brenda.
The detox strategy: vibrant health in 5 easy steps / Brenda Watson with Leonard Smith.
p. cm.
Includes bibliographical references and index.
1. Detoxification (Health) I. Smith, Leonard, 1942– II. Title.
RA784.5.W377 2008
613—dc22
2007043729

ISBN-13: 978-1-4165-7253-4
ISBN-10: 1-4165-7253-8
ISBN-13: 978-1-4165-7254-1 (pbk)
ISBN-10: 1-4165-7254-6 (pbk)

*For my husband, Stan, who shares my vision and
has supported me in bringing it to the world*

CONTENTS

THE
DETOX
STRATEGY

A TIME TO RENEW

❦

This is the most important book I will write in my career. In June 2006 the World Health Organization (WHO) reported that nearly one-quarter of global disease is caused by environmental exposures, but perhaps most striking is what it said next: "Well-targeted interventions can prevent much of this environmental risk," saving what could amount to millions of lives every year. This simple truth is the main reason I bring you The Detox Strategy: Vibrant Health in 5 Easy Steps. *I will give you an effective and practical plan for ridding your body and your life of harmful toxins that affect the vast majority of us today—including ones you may not know about hiding in unexpected places—so that you can achieve lifelong wellness.*

❦

Everyone deserves to feel as alive and energetic as possible, even if we do have to live with a few toxins that are an inevitable reality of our modern era. With this book I give you hope for a healthier tomorrow, and the promise that you can do something to support optimum health now and in the future. It will dispel myths you may have believed in the past about chemicals in our world and offer a revolutionary solution that will revitalize everything about you—body, mind, and spirit.

The subject of detoxification and cleansing has long been a source of controversy. When first I began cleansing it was considered "odd" or "strange" by many people. Yet, this healing philosophy has become much more accepted over the last ten years. Mainstream thought is just beginning to accept the fact that, as a society, we likely aren't detoxifying as well as we should. This is due to the overwhelming body of evidence about the dangers of toxicity, air and water pollution, and the buildup of chemicals in our environment—evidence that is mounting daily.

A cultural shift in the last few years alone has brought the topic of toxins to the forefront of the general public's attention, right alongside the issue of global warming. The two do, after all, go hand in hand in a lot of ways. We can no longer turn a blind eye to the onslaught of stories relating the insidious, long-lasting effects toxins can have on our bodies, on our planet, and the future of both. People increasingly seek the knowledge and secrets to leading healthy, robust lives. Who doesn't want to participate in life to the fullest, with abundant energy? Who doesn't want to avoid hospitals and a lifetime dependence on drugs? Now that science is catching up with proving the effects polluted environments can have on our quest for vibrant health, more and more people are ready to hear the message about toxins and ways to avoid them—or at least limit their impact—in everyday life. It's true that toxins can play a role in whether or not you can reach and maintain an ideal weight, whether or not you can bear and raise healthy children, and whether or not you would call yourself a happy person.

As I write this, reports are escalating about toxic toys coming from China. Recalls are in force and we are demanding new standards that will prevent such occurrences. Restaurants in major metropolitan areas are boycotting bottled water to help mitigate the damaging effects plastics have in the environment, where they cannot be broken down. (In addition, as you'll soon learn, plastics give off toxic chemicals that you then ingest when you—or your babies—drink from a bottle.) There's nothing more powerful than a collective voice for change. And I'm thrilled to be witnessing finally a growing united effort and interest in reducing the level of toxins in our lives.

My mission in teaching people how to live in a toxic world is a personal one. More than twenty years ago I was battling poor health, weight gain, and fatigue, and it was then that I discovered the natural healing principles that would ultimately change my life. I realized that by adopting a healthy diet and lifestyle—one that involved regular internal cleansing and detoxification—I could regain control of my body and my well-being. Since then it has become my passion to educate others and share with them the natural remedies that helped me achieve the superb health that I enjoy today. Upon dedicating my life to the fields of healthy digestion and detoxification, and to leading others onto the path of natural wellness, I have studied many philosophies of health and natural healing with some of the great teachers of our time. Through my work as a naturopathic doctor and founder of five natural health clinics in Florida that specialize in colon hydrotherapy and detoxification, I've watched people transform their lives in ways unimaginable to most who rely solely on traditional medicine or who think they must live with persistent illness, pain, and exhaustion.

During the past two decades I have watched the devastating effects of toxic exposure on the human body and the resulting decline in our overall digestive health because of the overwhelming number of chemicals to which we are exposed every day. Together these two factors have led to an alarming increase in chronic ailments, including cardiovascular disease, diabetes and obesity ("diobesity"), arthritis, depression, infertility, hormonal imbalances, allergies, gastrointestinal diseases, and cancer. In fact, the Centers for Disease Control (CDC) estimate that more than 90 million Americans live with chronic illness, and that "the prolonged course of illness and disability from such chronic diseases as diabetes and arthritis results in extended pain and suffering and decreased quality of life for millions of Americans." Causal links are also being found between toxins and autism, attention-deficit/hyperactivity disorder (ADHD), and developmental problems in children.

My first glimpse into the harsh reality of rising toxicity levels came as a result of working in a clinic for many years. There I observed the vast amount of people struggling to overcome disease, many of whom had finally come to the realization that in order to take control of their health, they needed to make significant changes to their diet and lifestyle—including their stress level. The biggest change of all, however, was the understanding that in order to establish a strong foundation of total-body wellness, they needed to fully comprehend the process of detoxification.

Without a doubt, the state of our planet's well-being, including its climate and ecosystems, has a measurable impact on our health, and that impact has prompted countless concerns about the level of toxicity that surrounds us each day and the ever-growing toxic burden with which our bodies must contend. Individuals, as well as health and government agencies, have begun to acknowledge this alarming reality and take steps to change it.

In its June 2006 report, titled "Preventing Disease Through Healthy Environments," the WHO focused on the environmental causes of disease

I once joked that we would someday be living in a "toxic soup" of dangerous chemicals, and now I realize how true those words were.

and how numerous diseases are influenced by environmental factors. In what is perhaps the most comprehensive study yet designed to examine how environmental factors, including exposure to unsafe water and indoor and outdoor air pollution, contribute to disease and ill health, the WHO stated that of the 102 major diseases reported yearly, 85 are partly caused by environmental factors, and it estimates that in the United States alone nearly 400,000 deaths each year are preventable simply by making improvements to our environment.

Having reported similar findings, the CDC feels so strongly about the connection between environmental factors and disease that they have created an entire department dedicated to the investigation of environmental exposure and disease. Over the last four years, the division of Environmental Hazards and Health Effects has laid the foundation for a national system designed to track environmental hazards and the diseases they cause. With the help of this system, dubbed the National Environmental Public Health Tracking Network, scientists, policymakers, communities, and the general public will soon have access to more information that they need to prevent exposure to the environmental factors that can lead to poor health and disease.

I once joked that we would someday be living in a "toxic soup" of dangerous chemicals, and now I realize how true those words were. As time has passed and the reports from health and governmental sources continue to corroborate my unintentional premonition, the future of our society's health has become disturbingly clear. The question is, What can we as individuals do to protect our own health and the health of our families in the coming years?

The purpose of this book is to provide information about the undeniable connection between environmental toxins and the health of the human body. But more than that, this book is a call to action for you to protect not only your health but also the future of our planet. I will show you how, and it's easier than you might think. It also doesn't require a serious investment of money or time. The biggest investment you will make is in taking in this knowledge. Applying it to your lifestyle will be relatively effortless. The payoff, however, can be huge.

Some of what you will learn may frighten you, but please don't let fear paralyze you from taking the steps starting today toward a healthier future. You will find many tried and true ideas on how to nourish and take care of yourself and your environment. You will also find that many techniques and strategies require only a slight shift from what you have already been doing. It's an easy-to-follow plan you can personalize for your life. My hope is that you take the knowledge in this book and become a change agent yourself—encouraging your loved ones and the people in your sphere of influence to adopt these principles of healthy living. Only then can we truly begin to change the world in which we live. Only then will the risk factors around us lessen as we do our part in creating a toxin-free world. This is not a gloom-and-doom treatise on chemicals and how they will ultimately bring on the end of human civilization. I write this book to inspire you, to motivate you, and to give you the gift of knowledge so that you can treat yourself to the gift of health.

While not a single day passes without someone's attempting to deny the need for regular internal cleansing and detoxification, this book will clearly explain why preserving the body's purification physiology is essential to achieving and maintaining the vibrant, lasting health you deserve. It begins with an eye-opening peek into the state of our toxic world, plus a test so you can gauge your personal level of toxic exposure. Then you complete Step 1: Reduce exposure to toxins in your environment.

I'll be taking you through your body's natural detoxification methods and help you to understand the ways in which you can support its functions through three sequential actions. Step 2 is to Eliminate toxins in your body via specific herbal cleansing regimens. In Step 3 you will Nourish your body properly to encourage optimal self-detoxification; and Energize (Step 4) through exercises and relaxation techniques designed to promote further the body's own health maintenance systems. I will give you formulas for jump-starting the cleansing process of your systems and explain how to replenish your cells with nutrients that will continue to foster good health. This completes the first four steps in the renewal process, which brings you to Step 5: Wellness. In the remaining chapters I will share more insights on where toxins come from, why, and the connection between chemicals and health as you begin your path to wellness. This is where you'll also find guidance on putting your entire RENEW program together in a sensible daily schedule. For continued support, updates, and online access to resources that will further assist you in this program, go to www.detoxstrategy.com.

If you want or require additional help in tailoring this program to your body, especially if you have any special health concerns or needs, please speak with your doctor. Your personal health practitioner can provide that extra guidance and individual support. I also encourage you to keep your doctor in the loop if you plan to commence an exercise program and have not been active in a while. Everyone's response to this program and results will be different.

By beginning this program and adopting a **RENEW**-based lifestyle, you are making a conscious choice: a choice to live a better, more fulfilling life. I can't think of a more profound decision to make, and I'm excited for you and the improved health that awaits you.

Your partner in optimum health,

Brenda Watson

CHAPTER 1

HOW TOXIC ARE YOU? TAKE THE TEST

❧

If you have been dealing with chronic illness, low energy, accelerated aging, or if you simply have had trouble losing unwanted fat, gaining mental clarity, and feeling the best and happiest you can, it's time for a change. And that change starts with an understanding of how toxic you are, where toxins come from, and what they potentially could be doing to you and your family from the inside out.

❧

When you look around and admire the comforts of modern life, chances are you don't recognize that many of our prized possessions and the things that make our life a *lifestyle* may be harboring silent killers. From common household goods that clean our bodies and countertops to our furniture, clothing, garden hoses, bottled waters, and favorite foods we think are nourishing us, known and unknown poisons lurk everywhere—and in lots of hidden, unexpected places.

We face a daily onslaught of chemicals that our bodies are not equipped to protect against sufficiently, and it's not surprising that for the first time in human history—in our lifetimes—we are witnessing unprecedented levels of degenerative illnesses and disorders such as cancer and heart disease, as well as the emergence of "new" ailments such as chronic fatigue syndrome, autism, and fibromyalgia. People are diagnosed with diseases at younger ages, and our children are now contracting chronic illness at alarming rates. Every day we seem to hear a study just published that links a health problem with a chemical or contaminant in our environment. Even our venerable medical community has had to admit to mistakes made in the creation of drugs that can be more harmful and toxic to people than the disease or disorder they are intended to treat.

So widespread and invasive are man-made substances (synthetics) in our world that I'm sorry to report, being alive on planet earth today tags us all with a label: toxic—guaranteed! The question is, how toxic are *you*? That's what we are going to answer in this first chapter. In doing so, you will begin to see just how pervasive, and often unavoidable, health-damaging substances are in our everyday life. Old theories about the effect they have on our bodies simply are not true: *The body can handle toxins—that's what the liver is for. The government will protect us from the really bad stuff. Increases in cancer and chronic disease are the result of people living longer and better detection techniques.* Sound familiar? These are among the most commonly held myths today.

The good news: you can do something starting today to live better, longer, to prevent future health problems, or turn your health around if it's been at a low point. Yes, toxins do exist, but so do ways to combat them. The techniques I give are practical, simple, and economical. As I explained in the Introduction, this book is not meant to stir up paranoia or give you the impression that the state of our toxic world is beyond your individual control. On the contrary, my main goal is to share the secrets to living healthier in a toxic world that you can adopt in your lifestyle. I will alert you to the common toxins you are most likely to encounter in your daily life and arm you with the knowledge to best avoid, limit, and manage their potentially harmful effects on your health, energy, and vitality. I will also show you how you can begin to change your environment through small-scale shifts, which can translate to large-scale transformations overall and revolutionize the quality of not only your life, but that of your children as well.

Even if you do just a fraction of the recommendations I offer, the benefits that await you could be tremendous. You will begin to think more clearly. You will feel sharper, stronger, and more alive. You may also notice physical changes in the mirror, from a better complexion to a smaller waistline. And you will likely sense that your body is simply happier. This is all in addition to the medical transformation that is taking place at the cellular level, where you stand a greater chance of combating disease and lowering your risk for future health problems. You may also find that you won't have to resort to or depend on drugs so much—both pharmaceutical and over-the-counter. With RENEW, you take a holistic approach to nurturing your body so it can continue to heal itself naturally no matter what it faces in day-to-day life.

YOUR BODY BURDEN

For decades scientists have been measuring the amount of industrial pollutants in air, water, and soil samples. Relatively new, however, is a biomonitoring process designed to measure what some experts refer to as our "body burden," or the level of toxins found in tissues of the human body, which involves the analysis of blood, urine, umbilical cord blood, and breast milk. Toxins are stored in most every tissue in the body ranging from fat, to cardiac and skeletal muscle to bones, tendons, joints, and ligaments, to visceral organs, and to the brain.

Recently a series of comprehensive studies intended to illustrate the human body burden has been conducted through the collaborative efforts of two nonprofit health and environmental research organizations: Environmental Working Group (EWG), based in Washington, D.C., and Commonweal, based in California. Both strive to use the power of communal information to contribute to and protect public and environmental health.

In 2000 EWG and Commonweal began the Human Toxome Project (HTP) to analyze human tissues for industrial chemicals that enter the body as pollution via food, air, and water, or from exposures to ingredients in everyday consumer products. Utilizing the latest technology, the project thus far includes a collection of seven studies involving 75 participants ranging in age from newborn to the elderly. Of those people, all 75 tested positive for a combined total of 455 out of 528 chemicals, including pesticides linked to birth defects and developmental delays; heavy metals shown to cause brain and nervous system disorders; and dangerous PCBs (polychlorinated biphenyls) that have been banned in the United States since 1977 because of their damaging effects on the skin, blood, urine, and liver. (For summaries of these findings, please refer to page 269 in the Notes.)

I believe these studies are just the tip of the iceberg, and our understanding of the long-term effects of toxic exposure in our increasingly noxious environment will grow. The actual number of chemicals contributing to our body burden is likely much higher than those investigated by the project. Our ability to identify toxins in the body is limited by what we know to look for, and how well we can find toxins based on current laboratory technology. Given the fact that many toxins hide deep in our tissues and tucked away in fat cells, I am prone to think we have much more to learn about this toxic library of possibilities. Uncovering how toxic exposure affects the human body is an emerging field of study that involves scientists, medical doctors, and engineers worldwide.

Also keep in mind that much of what we know about body burdens of contaminants comes from limited studies of a few contaminants, many of which are conducted by government agencies on selected groups of people. While these studies offer population-wide averages, they obviously cannot predict body burdens for individual people—and they cannot cover the gamut of all possible contaminants to which we are regularly exposed. Everyone reacts a little differently to chemicals, allergens, drugs, diseases, and external stimuli in general, which explains why the government's safety factors—including "safe" exposure limits for pollutants or contaminants in food and water—may not protect sensitive people.

Every citizen of an industrialized nation now carries an average of seven hundred synthetic chemicals in his or her body from food, water, and air—most of which have not been well studied.

Wombs Do Wound

Many experts once believed that the womb shielded the developing fetus from toxic exposure, but emerging evidence has proven otherwise. In actuality, the chemicals and pollutants to which the mother is exposed during her pregnancy are transferred from her bloodstream to that of her unborn child through the placenta. Not only has the Human Toxome Project demonstrated this when it found chemicals in cord blood and breast milk, but other studies also have proven that wombs are not safe havens from chemicals such as insecticides, pesticides, and heavy metals—some of the worst and most health-damaging toxins around. Toxic accumulation actually begins *before* birth. And it can last a lifetime.

Mercury, for example, is stored in the cardiac muscle in amounts 22,000 times greater than in skeletal muscle. During the aging process, as we experience low-grade inflammation and lose muscle mass, mercury (and other toxins) will get released into the bloodstream when those muscle cells shrink. Even the heart shrinks with aging. If the body is not equipped to handle that surfacing mercury efficiently through normal detoxification pathways, it will inflict more harm and intensify existing inflammation. Recirculating toxins may move into more critical areas like the brain and heart. As you can imagine, this will hasten the aging process.

DETERMINING YOUR PERSONAL BODY BURDEN

Different tests exist to help determine your individual body burden. You can, for instance, visit facilities that offer specialty testing to measure toxicity levels. These laboratories are usually CLIA certified by the Centers of Medicaid and Medicare Services, which regulate all laboratory testing performed on humans in the United States. They are dedicated to providing tests to health care providers, and typically analyze feces, hair, liver function, urine, and blood to arrive at a comprehensive conclusion. (For more specifics on these tests, see the list on pages 15-16.)

One such laboratory is Doctor's Data, Inc., based in Illinois. Offering a variety of tests to assess, detect, prevent, and even treat heavy metal burden, nutritional deficiencies, gastrointestinal function, and liver detoxification, Doctor's Data is a specialist and pioneer in essential and toxic elemental testing of multiple human tissues. Another very valuable service available to the general public is direct testing, through companies such as LabSafe.com and Labtestingdirect.com. These companies offer a large variety of laboratory testing, including forty-one different tests for toxins. These tests can range in cost from $79 to $359. (Please note that I am not affiliated with any of these labs, but have used them in the past and at this writing trust them to be reliable. You'll find information on these labs, plus other resources including government agencies and health care facilities in the Resource Directory.) Why can't you ask your family doctor for help? Unfortunately, your own physician is limited in the kinds of tests he can perform on you. Customary blood and urine tests will not necessarily detect a given toxin that's doing damage to you but remains "invisible." Many of today's toxic chemicals can hide under the radar of standard medical testing.

Moreover, most doctors are trained to treat symptoms and may not be well versed in the area of toxins and how they affect human health (especially if your doctor received his education decades ago). And when they do search for clues to an illness's origins, they routinely look for traditional causes such as an invading bacteria or virus, or, in the case of liver cirrhosis, drinking too much alcohol. Few doctors will investigate another potential genesis that relates to toxins, chiefly because they don't have the resources or know-how to do so. Textbook cases of illnesses attributed to toxins don't have a strong voice or foothold yet in conventional medical circles. That "textbook" is currently being written by pioneering scientists and doctors studying this burgeoning field of environmental medicine. As the evidence mounts, however, we will likely (and hopefully) watch the medical industry evolve. Newly trained doctors will gain experience in identifying and diagnosing illnesses based on the perspective that toxins could be partly or principally to blame.

I highly respect and value the expertise of medical doctors, but they are limited in how they can help you evaluate your body burden. As noted before, however, I recommend that you consult with your physician as you embark on this program and share with him or her your experience (and your results, if you do choose to go to a specialty laboratory). As with any program that involves your health, you should make this a team effort with your family physician. You may even bring new insights to your doctor and add value and knowledge to his practice that can then be passed on to other patients.

Specialty testing definitely has its merits, but it is not usually necessary unless you are dealing with serious health issues. A simple questionnaire like the one below will give you some idea.

LABS THAT CONDUCT SPECIALTY TESTING TO DETERMINE AN INDIVIDUAL'S BODY BURDEN WILL OFTEN ANALYZE THE FOLLOWING:

Feces Many toxic metals, such as mercury, cadmium, lead, antimony, and uranium, are eliminated primarily through the stool and can be detected there. This can also include dietary exposure to metal toxins.

Hair Hair may be dead cells, but it holds many keys that are indicators of toxic loads. As protein is synthesized in the hair follicle, elements get incorporated permanently into the hair—both toxic elements such as aluminum, arsenic, lead, and mercury, as well as essential ones such as calcium, magnesium, and potassium. Scalp hair is easy to sample, and because it grows an average of one to two centimeters a month, it contains a chronological record of your body's metabolism of certain elements and exposure to toxic ones. Remember, not all elements found in hair are bad. Nutrient elements including magnesium, chromium, zinc, copper, and selenium are necessary cofactors for hundreds of important enzymes and also are essential for the normal functions of vitamins. The levels of these elements in hair correlate to levels in organs and other tissues. Toxic elements, on the other hand, may be 200 to 300 times more highly concentrated in hair than in blood or urine.

Therefore, hair is often the tissue of choice for detection of recent exposure to elements such as arsenic, aluminum, cadmium, lead, antimony, and mercury. The CDC acknowledges the value of hair mercury levels as a maternal and infant marker for exposure to neurotoxic methyl mercury from fish. One caveat, however, is that hair is vulnerable to external elemental contamination by means of certain shampoos, bleaches, dyes, and curing or straightening treatments. So a first step in the interpretation of a hair element report is to rule out sources of external contamination.

Liver The body continually attempts to eliminate chemical toxins in the liver. By-products of liver functions are key indicators of chemical exposure, liver damage, and the capability of the liver to eliminate toxins. Some of these by-products are enzymes that can be detected in urine. For example, elevated levels of D-glucaric acid in urine indicate exposure to toxins such as pesticides, fungicides, petrochemicals, drugs, toluene, formaldehyde, and styrenes.

Urine Analysis of elements in urine provides diagnostic information on potentially toxic elements—lead, mercury, cadmium, nickel, beryllium, arsenic, and aluminum can be detected in urine. It can also help determine whether your kidneys are able to retain health-sustaining elements such as magnesium, calcium, sodium, and potassium.

Blood Separate analyses can be done to red blood cells, whole blood, and serum respectively to help determine a variety of element loads. For example, analysis of red blood cells provides the best diagnostic tool for assessing the status of elements that have important functions inside cells or on blood cell membranes. This is useful for evaluating cardiac influences, anti-inflammatory processes, anemia, immunological function, glucose tolerance, and other disorders that are associated specifically with zinc deficiency. Whole blood analysis measures total levels of elements that circulate in both extracellular fluids (serum/plasma) and in cells (red blood cells and lymphocytes). Some elements are measured in serum because they are transported by serum proteins, or have important extracellular functions in blood. The combination of the whole-blood analysis and the serum analysis provides a comprehensive evaluation of the status of elements. Source: Doctor's Data, Inc. ∎

THE BODY BURDEN TEST

Instructions: Read each question, and then check the box if you answer "yes."

- ❏ Do you brush your teeth daily?
- ❏ Do you have "silver" dental fillings?
- ❏ Have you ever had tooth extractions and/or root canal fillings?
- ❏ Do you use unfiltered tap water to brush your teeth, shower, make coffee or drink?
- ❏ Do you use commercial household cleaners, cosmetics or antiperspirants?
- ❏ Have you ever taken prescription medications or over-the-counter medications, including hormone replacement therapy or birth control?
- ❏ Do you have wall-to-wall carpet in your home or office?
- ❏ Do you eat commercial (non-organic) vegetables, fruits, or meat?
- ❏ Do you wear clothes that have been dry-cleaned?
- ❏ Do you wear synthetic materials (such as polyester)?
- ❏ Do you eat processed food or fast food?
- ❏ Have you ever smoked or been exposed to second-hand smoke?
- ❏ Do you eat in restaurants more than twice weekly?
- ❏ Do you use bug spray in your home or have a pest control service?
- ❏ Do you use weed killer on your lawn?
- ❏ Do you dye or bleach your hair?
- ❏ Do you use cologne or perfume?
- ❏ Are you overweight, underweight, or do you have cellulite deposits?
- ❏ Does your occupation expose you to toxins?
- ❏ Do you drink alcoholic beverages regularly?
- ❏ Do you eat fish more than twice a week?
- ❏ Do you regularly swim in a pool or lake?
- ❏ Do you live in a major metropolitan area?
- ❏ Do you live near an airport?
- ❏ Do you work in an environment using fluorescent lighting?
- ❏ Do you drink non-organic coffee?

❑   Do you feel tired, lethargic, or sluggish upon waking and even throughout the day?

❑   Do you have difficulty concentrating or have slow or surreal thinking?

❑   Do you feel depressed or have mood changes?

❑   Do you get more than one or two colds per year?

❑   Do you get postnasal drip, congestion, or a stuffy nose or sinuses upon waking or throughout the day?

❑   Do you have bad breath, a coated tongue, or a bitter or metallic taste in your mouth?

❑   Do you have strong body odor?

❑   Do you have strong-smelling urine?

❑   Do you have trouble sleeping or feel unrefreshed upon waking?

❑   Are your nails weak, soft, or brittle?

❑   Do you have dark circles under your eyes?

❑   Do you often feel stressed or anxious?

❑   Do you have allergies to various household products, dust, and molds?

❑   Do you have eczema, dry skin, acne, or rashes?

❑   Do you gain weight easily?

❑   Do you have food cravings, especially carbohydrate-rich foods and/or sweets?

❑   Do you have pain or discomfort on the right side of your stomach occasionally or after eating?

❑   Are you constipated or do you have less than one bowel movement per day?

Do you have any of the following symptoms:

❑   Sensitivity to perfume or other chemical odors

❑   Persistent joint and/or muscle pain

❑   Chronic infections

❑   Depression

❑   Fatigue

❑   Headaches

The higher your score, the greater the potential toxic burden you may be carrying and the more you may benefit from a detoxification program. (If you scored below 10, you are not living on planet earth in the twenty-first century, you have fibbed on the test, or you are living a very sheltered life!)

If you scored higher than 25: You are a prime candidate for completing the entire de-tox program from start to finish, beginning with the total-body basic cleanse and moving through the optional liver and heavy metal cleanses (these will be described in full detail in Chapter 5). Don't rush the program, by trying to do both the basic cleanse and heavy metal cleanse, for example, at once. Follow the sequence as recommended. It's important to take a slow, gradual approach. This will help you avoid possible cleansing reactions.

Cleansing is the process of cleaning out and reducing the toxic load that currently resides in your body. Because so many toxins hide beyond the bloodstream, the mere action of cleansing brings them out of hiding and dumps them into the bloodstream. When that happens, you can then "reexperience" the effect of those toxins all over again before they are flushed from the body. A cleansing reaction, also known as a Herxheimer reaction or a healing crisis, is the temporary physical discomfort that may result if toxins are released faster than your body can get rid of them. This can cause such symptoms as fever, fatigue, diarrhea, cramps, headache, increased thirst, appetite loss, flulike conditions, skin eruption or irritations. These reactions are generally short-lived, often lasting just a day or two, and usually no longer than a week. (Drug addicts who go through targeted programs for their particular substance abuse typically experience this reaction, and have been known to feel their highs all over again as those toxins come out.) Symptoms may range from mild to severe, depending upon the rate of cleansing.

Because you likely carry a heavier load of toxins than those who score lower, you'll avoid fasting and focus on making healthier choices at your meal times. My detox diet ideas will teach you how to start shifting your diet toward a cleaner lifestyle. I'll be giving specific instructions in Chapter 5 about how you can reduce the dosage of your supplement regimen if you do experience too many negative side effects and need to slow down the program further. (This usually only occurs during the targeted cleanses, chiefly the cleanse for heavy metals.) You are not likely to experience cleansing reactions on this program, as my recommended formulas are gentle and designed for both beginners (people who've never done a detox program before) and those familiar with the practice.

If you scored below 25: Aim to complete the entire program as recommended. However, you may also choose to do the three-day fast. If you scored low, you can further benefit by focusing on your diet more rigorously and cleaning out foods (and kicking out habits) that may have crept into your lifestyle. For example, if you've gotten into a habit of consuming sugary beverages and snacks in the late afternoon, you would do well to take notice of this and replace the habit with a nutritious juice blend or fiber bar. (Again, you'll find all the details and directions for creating a schedule for yourself in later chapters. I'll also be giving you plenty of ideas for meals and snacks that will help you fill your day with good nutrition and complement the detox process. Specific guidelines on how frequently you should be detoxing, and for how many days, will also be provided.)

Chapter 1 Summary

- The Human Toxome Project was designed to illustrate the effects of exposure to industrial chemicals on the human body by testing the blood, urine, breast milk, and other tissues of selected participants.

- Studies have shown that toxic exposure begins in the womb, since the developing fetus is exposed to the toxins in its mother's blood through the placenta.

- A quick self-test can help you gauge your personal body burden.

- For those who want a full report on their body burden, specialty tests at various labs throughout the country can help determine your personal body burden. Unless you have a serious medical issue, you can simply answer a few questions to gauge your level of toxicity. This will then help you begin to focus on areas in your life and lifestyle that need to be cleaned up!

- Whether you score low or high on the body burden test, you can benefit by going through the detox program from start to finish. This program is designed for those who likely bear a lot of toxins and have never gone through a detoxification program before, as well as those who lead relatively healthy lives but want to focus on upping their health quotient even more.

CHAPTER 2

THE PERILS OF POLLUTANTS AND THE POWER OF DETOXIFICATION

❧

When we think of pollution, visions of factories belching out toxic gases from their smokestacks are likely to come to mind. The industrial age has proven to be a mixed blessing. On the one hand, it has brought technology, innovation, and convenience, and on the other, it has liberated unprecedented amounts of toxic substances into our air, water, and soil— which can land in the farthest reaches of the earth. But bear in mind that classic images of pollution can perpetuate myths about who is exposed to what. You don't have to live near a factory or in a city to feel the effects of pollution. It's a global problem. Americans inhale fumes from Asia, as the winds and currents push our waste toward Europe. Even the earth's poles cannot hide from pollution's insidious effects.

❧

A great deal of environmental damage was done before we began monitoring and attempting to control pollution. But even though we acknowledged a growing problem, we have not yet found a way to eliminate the release of so many toxins. Current technology can only reduce them. The United States Environmental Protection Agency (EPA) periodically releases a report called the Toxics Release Inventory. The EPA annually collects information on the disposal or other releases and other waste management activities for more than 650 chemicals from industrial sources in all 50 states. For 2005, the latest data collected, disposal and releases of these chemicals totaled nearly 4.34 billion pounds from almost 23,500 United States facilities. This report shows that 1.51 billion pounds of chemicals where released via air emissions, 787 million pounds of chemicals were deposited into waste dumps, 626 million pounds of chemicals injected into underground wells, and 596 million pounds of chemicals were released into our environment via other land disposal such as spills or leaks. This discharge of chemicals impacts not only Americans, but every single person on all seven continents. Through studies done by the National Institutes of Health, we now have reason to believe that as many as two-thirds of *all* cancer cases may be linked to environmental causes.

The Toxic Hit List

drugs

heavy elements and metals

household chemicals and solvents

infections

herbicides and pesticides

alcohol

air pollution

tobacco

water pollution

caffeine

"THINK GLOBALLY, ACT LOCALLY"

Today's concerns with regard to global warming as a result of a stronger greenhouse effect (the rise in the earth's temperature when certain gases in the atmosphere trap energy from the sun) highlight the negative planetary effects of large-scale industrial production. The greenhouse effect is a normal part of earth-sun dynamics; without it the earth would be too cold for humans (and many other species) to live. Certain gases in the atmosphere, including water vapor, carbon dioxide, nitrous oxide, and methane, trap heat from the sun to keep the earth warm. But when we enhance this effect, we risk making the planet warmer than usual, which can have potentially devastating consequences. These concerns magnify with every report of oil spills, disappearance of rain forests, species extinctions, and so on. For some people, the "Save the Planet" mantra sounds like a monumental mission for the individual; but if you simply think small-scale—if you merely live with a "Save the Body" mentality—you will be doing your part in the global quest for a healthier, cleaner world. And that can be a very motivating, deeply satisfying way of thinking. You can't get much more local than focusing on your own body, and it may just be the best way to start effecting change in our world at large. The bonus, of course, is the physical rejuvenation you will experience in doing so.

Another way to envision the magnitude of our society's industrial waste—besides the numbers of how much gets disposed of or released into the environment annually—is to know that industry currently uses between 75,000 and 100,000 chemicals, with an additional 1,000 introduced each year. These include everything from flame-retardant furniture and fabric coatings to polycarbonate plastics. The health effects of very few of these (less than 10 percent) have been tested, so there are no data to suggest that they are safe—and remarkably few regulatory procedures put into place to ensure that they are not. The Toxic Substances Control Act (TSCA), enacted by Congress in 1976, gives the United States Environmental Protection Agency (EPA) "broad authority to identify and control substances that may pose a threat to human health or the environment." And even with such standards in place there are loopholes. For example, certain chemicals already in commerce prior to and even *after* the enactment of TSCA do not require testing, regardless of whether or not they may cause harm.

One of the chief concerns with toxins in the environment is the fact we are at the top of the food chain and are more likely to be exposed to an accumulation of toxic substances in the food supply (often called "bioaccumulation"). Grains sprayed with pesticides, for instance, are then fed to animals that store those toxic substances in their fatty tissue. The animals also store other toxins such as hormones, antibiotics, and other chemicals administered by farmers. When people eat these products, they are exposed

FACT

Our body naturally tries to eliminate these toxins, but overexposure to any or all of these will slow down or even damage our body's systems, including its capacity to detoxify on its own.

to the full range of chemicals and additives that have been used along the entire agricultural chain. The increased incidence of children, for example, who experience puberty early (before the age of ten), has been blamed partly on abnormal exposure to hormones. "Precocious puberty," as it is called, can happen because of foods such as chicken and milk that contain added hormones. Bioaccumulation of toxic substances over time is responsible for many physical and mental disorders, especially ones that are on a rapid rise such as asthma, cancer, and mental illness. It's no surprise that as a result, detoxification therapies are increasing in importance and popularity.

More than a Food Chain: As you can see in this illustration, our world is interconnected far beyond simple food-chain dynamics. We are consumers *and* producers of products that share the same environment.

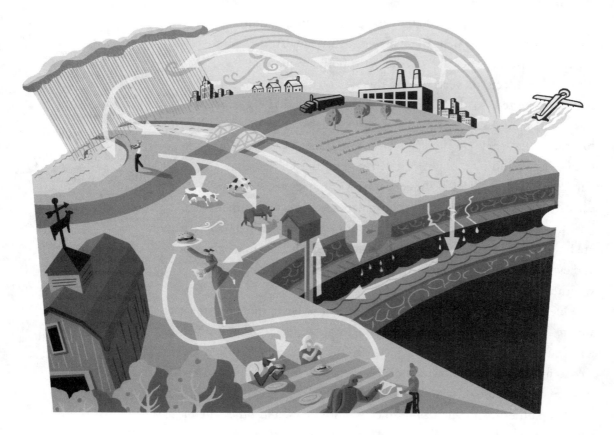

WHAT QUALIFIES
AS A TOXIN?

It helps to first examine what the very word *toxin* means. Traditionally, by definition, a toxin is "a poisonous substance," as the word has its roots in the Greek word *toxikon,* which literally translates into "poison." Today the term is used to describe anything that is foreign or poisonous to the body. Although we can certainly have toxic relatives and relationships, I generally use the term to discuss two broad classes: environmental and internal. Environmental toxins include household chemicals, industrial pollutants, food additives, and pesticides. Internal toxins consist of waste products created by normal metabolic processes within the body. Such digestive toxins are produced as a result of breaking down proteins, carbohydrates, and fats.

But I also want to point out another dimension to this definition that's frequently overlooked. Substances you wouldn't normally view as "toxic" or "poisonous" are indeed members of this category. These include pharmaceutical drugs, caffeine, and alcohol. The number of people who died in 2001 as a result of conditions brought on inadvertently by either medical treatment or diagnostic procedures was greater than the number of those who died in that same year of either heart disease or cancer, the number one and two leading causes of death in the United States respectively. Moreover, deaths or injuries related to drug treatments more than doubled between 1998 and 2005 in this country, with painkillers and immune-system boosters accounting for most. (For more on this topic, see Appendix C.)

So even if you think aspirin, coffee, and red wine are benefiting you, from a purely technical standpoint they are toxins by virtue of the fact they are foreign substances that your body, and especially your liver, has to process. Obviously, there may be a time and place for these substances, and it's important to note that not all "toxins" are bad at all times. But I want you to get used to this word, and understand that detoxification aims to return the body to a more natural state, in which it is minimally bombarded by the toxins that can downgrade your health and put you on a path to physical, emotional, and spiritual illness.

This is why I call my program RENEW—it's a way to literally renew the body. While activists continue to push for changes such as reducing the pesticides in foods, higher standards for our air and drinking water, and tougher standards for heavy metal exposure, my prescription focuses on what you can do right now as an individual. So much that's out there currently is about what you should *not* do; RENEW emphasizes the healthful solutions you can follow, and the positive things you *can* do for your family, your home, and yourself.

WHAT IS DETOXIFICATION?

While the word *detoxification* may conjure images of drugged-out celebrities in rehab for substance abuse, from a scientific perspective it actually refers primarily to the body's natural methods of self-cleansing—of ridding wastes that are the by-products of its normal function, and dealing with potentially harmful invaders such as bacteria, viruses, or toxic chemicals. Detoxification is a constant bodily process. We are continually eliminating excess toxins through our digestive, urinary, skin, circulatory, respiratory, and lymphatic systems. A secondary meaning of the word relates to the treatments and concepts employed by medicine to help support the structure and function of these natural detoxification channels, which you will learn about in Chapter 4. Detoxification in this sense is about taking an active role in stimulating your body's innate ability to cleanse itself.

Many people view detoxification in a very narrow sense, seeing it as synonymous with colon cleansing. And when asked, most people will define "cleansing" as increased bowel elimination or just colon cleansing, and they think they will have to take a laxative, stay home from work, and sit by the bathroom. This is not the case, as the colon is just one of many channels of elimination. Because toxins are present throughout the body, detoxification (which includes cleansing) cannot be limited to just bowel cleansing—and you won't have to camp out in the bathroom for a month. These regimens are gentle and will detoxify in a gradual, steady process without disruptive side effects. Detoxification must be viewed as a total-body process for all of the body's organ systems. It is as much a series of actionable steps as it is a set of daily habits that becomes a lifestyle.

For purposes of this book, when I refer to "detoxification" I am referring to the act of supporting your body's innate detox methods as well as renewing your body in its totality through specific cleansing regimens and attention to diet and exercise. The goal is to enhance or improve your overall health and give your body what it craves to remain toxin free and in peak condition for life. The specific actions and recommendations to achieve this are the heart and soul of the RENEW program. It works with the body's own systems of self-healing to strengthen every tissue and enhance the overall functions of every part. It's noninvasive, and rooted in an understanding of the body's intrinsic capacity to recapture health in the face of injury or illness.

Because detoxification is based on the body's natural rehabilitative faculties, it is very effective for a wide variety of health problems, as well as being safe and helpful for virtually everyone.

A Little History

Contrary to what you might think, detoxification methods of healing have been used across all cultures for centuries. They are not an invention of new age medicine. Fasting, for example, is one of the oldest therapeutic practices in medicine. In fact, internal detoxification and cleansing are as old as the idea of health. Four thousand years ago, according to the earliest medical textbook ever discovered (the Ebers Papyrus, found in the sands of Egypt), physicians were already using enemas to help the body cleanse and fight off disease. Around the year 400 BCE, Hippocrates, the Greek doctor generally accepted as the father of Western medicine, gave his patients cleansing herbs to help their bodies heal and was an advocate of fasting for improved health. Galen, another highly influential Greek physician, born 129 CE, believed cleansing was crucial to keeping the body in balance and good health. Ayurvedic medicine, a traditional healing system that has developed over thousands of years, utilizes detoxification methods to treat many chronic conditions and to prevent illness.

It's very empowering to know we can reduce our risk for disease and lessen our exposure to these ubiquitous toxins that are a product of our modern culture and, inevitably, our attempts to advance the science of food, agriculture, medicine, and engineering in general. Our diets and health are unfortunately largely controlled by three giant sectors and driving forces of the economy: food and agricultural corporations, including processed food giants; pharmaceutical companies; and the chemical and manufacturing industry, which aims to create unnaturally occurring products that may be superior in some ways to naturally occurring ones, yet incredibly harmful to humans in other ways. Because these three sectors are huge economic generators, we are led to believe their activities are okay—that processed and chemically altered or modified foods and agriculture, as well as chemically engineered goods and drugs, are actually better than what nature would provide. But this is far from the truth. They may be better in the sense that they make our lives easier, but the cost is exposure to potentially harmful substances.

Many of the toxins you will read about in this book are so foreign to us that we simply cannot detoxify efficiently through breathing and sweating, for instance. The necessity of proper detoxification and cleansing is reinforced for me every day as I listen to people express their gratitude for finding solutions to living in a toxic world and nurturing their bodies as best they can through the RENEW techniques. They share their joy about feeling like a whole new person. And that is my hope for you, too.

THE SKINNY ON FAT-LOVING TOXINS

The skull and crossbones is widely known as the universal symbol for toxicity, yet not all toxic substances are labeled in this manner—if they are labeled at all. While a container of a highly toxic substance, such as lead or arsenic, will likely bear the skull and crossbones symbol, another substance, such as drinking water, which may contain trace amounts of these toxins, will not be so marked. Likewise, even though the can of insect spray beneath your counter will include a warning on the label, the strawberries you purchased from your local supermarket will not, despite the fact that they may contain trace amounts of the same (or related) toxic compounds (a result of pesticide application to commercially grown crops).

In fact, myriad products we use daily can harbor toxic substances that our bodies absorb little by little over time—from mattresses, magazines, and mouthwash to carpets, clothing, and cosmetics. (For a provocative yet alarming tour from the moment you step out of bed in the morning, see Chapter 9.) We may worry about our children falling from playground equipment and injuring themselves, but we should be more concerned about toxic levels of arsenic coming off treated wood in playground equipment. Children are more likely to be exposed to harmful levels of arsenic from play structures, picnic tables, and decks than from drinking water. In addition, other preservatives applied to the equipment so that it can withstand the outdoor elements, including chromium, copper, and pentachlorophenol (penta, or PCP for short) may also pose a serious health threat to children sensitive to these chemicals.

Because each one of us is encoded with a unique DNA, each person has a unique response to chemical toxins. We are now at the place in clinical medicine where the evaluation of genes and mutations are becoming more useful in predicting who will have toxicity issues even with minimal exposures. In the near future we may see a rising demand for all fetal and newborn children to have amniotic fluid and blood testing for genetic mutations that can result in higher levels of toxicity. This type of testing can give important information on what type of lifestyle, diet, and supplements the pregnant mother and infant should take to optimize their health and avoid the nutritional and toxic disasters that can face unborn children and infants. Let me give you an example.

As many as 10 percent of Caucasians produce low levels of a specific enzyme required for proper detoxification in the body. In fact, at least twenty-five commonly used drugs need this enzyme to be present in the body for the detox pathway to work efficiently. So it's easy to see if this enzyme is low and the person is, let's say, taking Prozac for depression, the possibility of Prozac overdose becomes a real one. This is especially true if the person has significant toxin exposure (as most of us do). It's also well known in the medical community that excessively elevated serotonin levels (from Prozac or other SSRIs) can cause suicidal depression the same way too low of a level of serotonin can. Which begs the question: Could some of the suicides blamed on these antidepressants have been prevented with simple genetic testing for the gene that's responsible for the detox enzyme? I personally think so.

Interestingly, on the other hand, some folks make *too much* of this enzyme (as well as other enzymes) and require *higher* doses of drugs for the therapeutic benefit. These may be the same people who live long and with relatively unhealthy lifestyles! (Yet another reason to consider genetic testing as it becomes more available to see how many degrees of freedom you may have in the direction of toxicity.) I think these examples, of which there are thousands now, will encourage more genetic testing in the future for practicing good medicine, age management, and detoxification. Hopefully it will soon become a medical standard of care. (For more details see Genova Diagnostics in the Resource Directory and the *Textbook of Functional Medicine*, at www.functionalmedicine.org.)

Obviously, the higher the exposure to a certain toxin or toxins, the more symptoms of the illness the body will manifest and the more immediate, or acute, the response will be. But what happens when the dose to which we are exposed is so small as to cause no immediate symptoms? Does this mean there is no harm done? Not necessarily. Many chemicals are slowly deposited in our bodies where they may remain, build up over time, and do lasting damage. It is for this reason that professionals in natural health care place a heavy emphasis on toxicity as a major cause of disease. What's more, no matter how toxins get into our bodies—through the lungs, stomach, or skin—they all meet the liver at some point and from there, get sent to the kidneys and colon for eliminating, become stored away in fat cells, trapped in bones, muscles, tissues, and organs, or get locked up in the liver itself.

The fact that many toxins can park themselves in fat cells deserves special attention. Fat cells don't get broken down easily and sit like cargo bins weighing the body down physically. This is troubling news given the rising rates of obesity in the world. If you carry excess fat, you have to burn up those fat cells to release fat-residing toxins into the bloodstream for proper removal. We all know how difficult weight loss can be, so this presents an added challenge. In addition, toxins being released from fat stores may slow the thyroid down, a pivotal gland in regulating metabolism. When the thyroid slows down, so does your metabolism—leading to weight gain and low energy. As the toxins accumulate, they eventually eke out in unexpected ways. You begin to experience health problems, from minor ones like allergies and endless colds, to migraines and infertility, to full-throttle illnesses such as incurable cancer and dementia.

Avoiding the fat-soluble toxins may sound like a solution, but that's difficult to do today. We have considerable exposure to fat-soluble, carbon-containing, toxic chemicals used as solvents, glues, and paints. Common cleaning products, formaldehyde, toluene, and benzene are all solvents (meaning they are capable of dissolving other substances) we can typically encounter in daily life when we pump gas, shop for clothes, buy a new car, and pick up laundry. These fat-soluble chemicals collect in the fatty tissues of the body rather than being excreted quickly. They are particularly damaging to those who are deficient in essential fatty acids, because a body deprived of essential fats is a body that will grab onto oily substances—even if that includes toxic substances like diesel fuel—just as a dry sponge readily soaks up water. These compounds can cause liver and kidney damage, as well as skin irritation, which brings me to a note about weight I want to highlight.

FACT
According to some reports, at death the human body decomposes more slowly today than just thirty years ago, thanks to all those preservatives and synthetic chemicals absorbed.

Detox and Weight Loss

Of all the benefits that a detoxification program and subsequent healthier lifestyle provides, achieving and maintaining an ideal weight routinely ranks high on people's lists. It's important to understand that several factors contribute to weight gain, two of which are the combination of toxins and a faulty diet. Both of these can create a condition in the body by which you become insulin resistant—your cells become desensitized to insulin, making them ineffective at driving blood sugar (glucose) into your cells. Insulin is a hormone secreted by the pancreas in response to a meal; its job is to unlock your tissues and escort glucose out of the blood into the tissue cells for use as energy.

When excess glucose remains in the blood, insulin levels stay high. Even though the right amount of insulin is essential for life, chronically elevated insulin can cause both fat storage and more inflammation, which can promote even more fat storage. Because detox programs entail a high-quality diet, hydration, exercise, and proper elimination, blood sugar balance is achieved, normalizing insulin levels, decreasing inflammation, and helping one to lose fat!

In Dr. Mark Hyman's *Ultrametabolism: The Simple Plan for Automatic Weight Loss,* he calls for detoxifying the liver as a critical step to weight loss, pointing to the fact that a healthy functioning liver makes for a healthy functioning metabolism that can properly process sugars and fats. He underscores that toxins from within our bodies and from our environment both contribute to obesity. So getting rid of toxins and boosting your natural detoxification system is an essential component of long-term weight loss and a healthy metabolism. I couldn't agree with him more.

FACT

A Vicious Cycle: The more fat you have, the more toxins you retain. The more toxins you retain, the harder it becomes to lose weight. A simple solution: Minimize your exposure to toxins in your environment and lifestyle, and remove toxins from your body through proper detoxification methods.

In particular, toxins can impact your ability to achieve an ideal weight in three big ways: slowing down your metabolism, decreasing your ability to burn fat, and slowing down the time it takes for you to feel full.

In the past it was thought that your resting metabolic rate (RMR) declined with weight loss primarily because of the decrease in caloric intake or changes in muscle to fat ratio. But clinical studies are now showing that one of the first things toxins do when your fat cells release them into the blood is *slow down* your resting metabolic rate. Moreover, the same studies determine that toxins affect the production of the thyroid hormones, which as I just mentioned play a major role in your body's metabolism.

What this means is that if you can reduce your exposure to toxins while aiding in the elimination of current toxins in your body, you can support a healthy—and possibly faster—metabolism. Don't worry about any potential slowdown in your metabolism during the actual detoxification process. In all likelihood, you will be eliminating toxins from your body fast enough to prevent much of this decline. If you do experience this, it will be very temporary and you may not even notice it. Chances are your weight is going to tick downward given the metabolism-revving foods you will be eating as you nourish your cells and follow the recommendations of the diet.

For thirty years now we've known that toxins can hinder the efficiency of your fat-burning systems—by upwards of 20 percent! On a hormonal level, toxins stored in our fat cells can prevent us from receiving signals that tell our brains we are full so we can stop eating. Contrary to popular belief, fat cells are not inactive. Our total body fat mass may actually represent our *largest endocrine (hormonal) organ,* since it is much larger than our chief hormone-producing and -regulating organs—the pituitary, adrenal, thyroid, and sex glands. Fat generates a multitude of biomolecules—enzymes, hormones, and chemical messengers—that tell our bodies what to do, which in turn affects how we look and feel. This also affects our metabolism and whether it's running high or low.

Many of these molecules, including estrogen, cortisol, and leptin, can promote more fat storage. The aromatase enzyme in fat, for example, converts testosterone into estrogen and further promotes fat storage. The stress hormone cortisol is famous for its fat-promoting capabilities. Chronic elevation of this hormone raises blood sugar, increases insulin (which again increases fat storage), breaks down muscle, and blocks the conversion of thyroid hormone T4 to T3. Triiodothyrosine, or T3, is the biologically active thyroid hormone that moves into the nucleus of cells and affects the production of proteins critical to the mitochondria, which are the power generators of cells. So low T3 equals low energy, low metabolism, and more potential fat storage. This list goes on and on with similar scenarios in the body. In fact, much of what fat does is to continually signal the body to make more fat cells and store more energy via fat. In this process toxins are stored in fat as well, which then aggravate the situation even more by promoting *more* fat storage. These toxins essentially mess with the proper signaling we need for maintaining a good fat-to-muscle ratio. Other factors can also contribute to the chaotic signaling. Our 24/7 lives, where the lights are always on, we sleep rarely (and poorly), and we have an abundance of refined sugar available to keep us artificially charged, exacerbate the imbalance we experience in our body's internal workings. So it's a vicious cycle: the more fat you have, the more toxins you retain, and the more toxins you retain, the harder it becomes to lose weight as cascading events sabotage your metabolism. One way to end it is with proper detoxification, removing toxins from your environment as best you can, and adopting a lifestyle attuned to supporting your body's natural detox physiology. That's exactly what we are doing with the RENEW program. Through the detox program, you will be shrinking those fat cells, releasing stored toxins, and helping your body achieve not only an ideal weight but also an ideal balance of hormones and other metabolism-regulating substances that will further support vibrant health, energy, and longevity.

FACT

Toxins Trigger Water and Fat Retention: When faced with toxicity, which provides inflammation, our bodies respond by retaining water in an effort to dilute both fat-soluble and water-soluble toxins.

SILENT KILLERS

To get a quick understanding of the scope environmental toxicity has on widespread sickness and disease, a glimpse at the World Health Organization's numbers from its gathering of information and studies is shocking. It estimates that more than 13 million deaths each year are the result of environmental causes and could be prevented by taking steps toward decreasing global pollution. As I stated in the Introduction, of the 102 diseases regularly included in the WHO's annual assessment of global health (called *The World Health Report*), 85 are now known to be partially caused by exposure to environmental factors. The major ones, shown to have the largest impact on the environment in terms of death, illness, or disability, are as follows:

- **Diarrhea: 58 million incidences a year caused by environmental factors, primarily the result of unsafe water, sanitation, or hygiene**

- **Lower respiratory infections: 37 million incidences each year, or 41 percent of all cases globally, primarily caused by indoor and outdoor air pollution**

- **Chronic obstructive pulmonary disease (COPD): 12 million cases per year, or 42 percent, of all cases globally as a result of exposure to workplace contaminants, chemical fumes, and indoor and outdoor air pollution**

The WHO further states that most of the environmentally triggered diseases rank as the biggest killers outright. Below are the diseases with the largest absolute number of deaths annually from environmental factors:

- **Cardiovascular disease: 2.6 million deaths each year**
- **Diarrheal disease: 1.7 million deaths each year**
- **Lower respiratory infections: 1.5 million deaths each year**
- **Cancer: 1.4 million deaths each year**
- **COPD: 1.3 million deaths each year**

If you are having trouble understanding the link between toxins and most of these diseases, you will grasp the connections by the end of this book. They are astounding. Common knowledge may have you believe, for example, that heart disease is largely genetic, or the result of poor diet and lack of exercise. While those do factor into anyone's risk for developing heart disease, toxic metals such as arsenic, lead, and mercury are also strongly implicated in triggering heart disease. Halogens like chloride and fluoride, substances we are all regularly exposed to either in a simple compound or as part of a more complex, synthetic chemical, activate abnormal heart rhythms. Examples of halogen sources include gasoline, disinfectants and cleaning solutions, toothpaste, dyes, and medicines. Most drugs, in fact, are made with chlorine (you'll see the "Cl" in drug labeling).

It's been said that you absorb the vast majority of the sun's damage to your skin by the time you reach the ripe old age of eighteen. Well, it has also been suggested that by the time you were *six months old*, you had already absorbed about 30 percent of your total lifetime toxic load of chemicals. Some of that chemical load is largely due to the combinations of vaccines children receive that also contain additives. The mercury-based preservative thimerosal (brand name Merthiolate), for example, was removed as a health threat in 2001, but was a source of toxic mercury for millions of kids who received up to nine shots with this additive between 1988 and 2001. Thimerosal is still in some flu shots, and it's a hotly contested debate in political and medical circles. Other additives common in vaccines include aluminum, formaldehyde, monosodium glutamate (MSG), sulfites, and the antifreeze ingredient ethylene glycol. Each of these chemicals has been linked to a host of health issues, from ADHD to brain, cardiovascular, and metabolic disorders.

Throughout this book, and in particular chapters 9 and 10, you will learn about similar associations between toxins and disease. Many might surprise you, as will the truth to where poisons can loiter. Regardless of whether they are from environmental pollution, prescription or illegal drugs, synthetics, and various chemicals nature never intended us to ingest, all toxins harm the body to some degree. They create a heavy burden, triggering a general dysfunction of major systems and body chemistry. Because toxins generally impair the body's ability to function normally, they can be an underlying cause of fatigue, headaches, hormonal imbalances, mood swings, depression, muscle and joint pain, skin conditions, brain fog, problems thinking clearly, neurological dysfunction, low immunity, and much more. This, in turn, opens the door wide open to endless and sometimes life-threatening illness.

Side Effects and Signs of Toxicity

In addition to the self-test in Chapter 1, another way to gauge your toxicity level is to consider some of the side effects of toxins that can become chronic health problems. Below is a list; check off those that apply to you. Though you can't assume all of the following are attributed directly to toxins in your body, it helps to take stock of your health issues now so you can see if the RENEW program diminishes or even eliminates any of these conditions. (You may also want to be thinking about your family members as you read this list.)

acne

allergies

anxiety

arthritis

asthma

attention–deficit/ hyperactivity disorder (ADHD)

autism

autoimmune disorders

behavioral problems

bloating, belching, or intestinal gas

body odor

brain disease

cancer

cardiovascular disease

chronic or unexplained fatigue

chronic infections

colitis

connective tissue disorders

constipation

dementia

depression

diabetes

digestive problems

diarrhea

epilepsy

fibroid tumors

fibromyalgia

food allergies

frequent mood swings

general malaise or low energy

hayfever

headaches

high blood pressure

high cholesterol

hives

hormonal imbalances

hypertension

impotence

inability to concentrate

indigestion

infertility

inflammatory disorders

insomnia

irritable bowel syndrome

joint aches

memory lapses

migraines

mouth sores

multiple sclerosis

muscle pain

nausea

neuropsychiatric (mental) illness

obesity

Parkinson's disease

peptic ulcer

peripheral neuropathies

pigmentation

poor posture

potbelly

schizophrenia

seizures

skin rashes or disorders

sore throat

spastic colon

stroke

weight maintenance issues

THE POWER OF DETOXIFICATION

Don't panic if you "failed" the questionnaire and circled several of the health issues listed above. Toxins may not be the root cause of many of these illnesses so I don't want you to think that all health challenges relate directly to toxicity or that this detox program will guarantee that you are cured of a particular ailment. The purpose of this list is to show you how pervasive toxins can be in their effects on health across the broad spectrum of potential illnesses.

We can no longer pretend it's not real, and we can't ignore the reality that we live in a toxic world. But, more important, we can't ignore the fact *we can do something about it*. In my RENEW program I will show you exactly which choices can reduce your toxic exposure and remove the toxic residue from your body to improve the state of your health and up the quality of your life.

It's unrealistic to think we can totally eliminate all the toxic substances in the world and their risk factors. And, in some cases, even when we do, we may still experience side effects for years to come. Or we may have to endure years of a certain toxin's remnants that nature cannot eradicate the same day we decide to evict it from our lives. Toxic chemicals can remain in the environment and in our bodies for years, sometimes decades, after we've stopped manufacturing and using them. The best we can do is limit and manage our risks—without driving ourselves crazy or moving to Montana (forewarning: moving out of the city won't be your saving grace). Although many plastics can be among the most harmful creations of the modern era, this doesn't mean you have to stop touching and using all forms of plastic. We have to maintain some semblance of realism.

I'm not asking you to give up your job and start picketing outside your local waste site; change can start with you in simply the choices you make in your regular daily life.

You probably know that I've been in the digestive health field for many years, and I've watched people transform their lives through good nutrition, supplementation, and small shifts in their lifestyle to support a healthy body. As a champion of health and crusader for finding the secrets to optimum well-being, I can't express how powerful detoxification can be for addressing (and sometimes curing) common and even not-so-common ailments that can be rooted in toxin overload. I am especially committed to helping people cope with chronic diseases, which are the leading causes of morbidity and mortality in the United States. A limited number of health risk behaviors, such as cigarette smoking, poor nutrition, physical inactivity, and underuse of prevention practices, are linked to chronic diseases. But as the evidence mounts on the contribution of toxins to the progression and sustainability of chronic disease, there is a call to action. I continue to be amazed by how effective a detoxification program can be for a person—even someone who didn't think he or she was "toxic" and who doesn't have any specific health concern.

Think of detoxification as a way of giving your body the equipment it needs to act effectively as its own shield against these incoming toxins, many of which we just cannot circumvent today. Detoxification helps fuel the engines that will literally clean up your body at a cellular level and support its natural operations. It also can physically reboot your body so you can begin to make those little but transformational shifts in your lifestyle that will help you to live a richer, more energetic life. You *can* reverse the effects of aging and feel younger than ever before, no matter how old you are now.

Adopting a "healthy" lifestyle for some people is a challenge. But by going through a specific detox program first, you set the tone and give yourself a much-needed launching pad. You can then live a healthy lifestyle effortlessly day in and day out without feeling deprived. Your body will continue on its path to optimum wellness. And you will rarely again get "caught off guard" when it comes to your health or you read a headline in the paper about tainted tap water in your community.

We have become a society that no longer has to worry so much about things like plague, famine, and poor sanitation. We now suffer from the products and *by*-products of our own technological advancements that provoke poor health and chronic illness. In addition to ubiquitous chemical toxins, we have too much food, especially from unnatural, processed sources; we are oversanitized; and we owe our major health threats such as cancer, diabetes, and heart disease largely to lifestyle choices. These lifestyle choices, encompassing diet, exercise, consumerism, and stress management, perpetuate a vicious cycle of blows to our health. It also leaves us looking older, feeling more tired, and unable to do the things we want to do in life. Which is why I'm redefining "lifestyle" with easy, practical solutions that won't require radical change. I want you to beat the odds and live the best life.

GET READY TO RENEW

Of all the possible diseases we can get, cancer is the one that I find people are most perplexed about (and you'll find a lengthier discussion of cancer and its ties to toxins in Appendix B).

We see warnings all the time that substances "may cause cancer," and if and when we hear about a cancer diagnosis in our families or in ourselves, we naturally focus on the tumor itself. Thousands of studies prove the links between cancer and toxins, even though we may not have all the answers yet about how cancer starts or how we can stop it dead. The body is a puzzling piece of machinery. A substance doesn't necessarily have to be a "carcinogen" to have a toxic effect somewhere that eventually manifests itself as cancer somewhere else. This is why the focus needs to be on detoxification for the benefit of the body as a whole—as a unit beautifully made up of interwoven and interacting parts. If you detoxify and decrease your chances of getting cancer, guess what: you'll simultaneously increase your chances of achieving so much more. Ideal weight. Abundant energy. Sound sleep. Beautiful skin. A sharp mind. Vibrant general health that can defy your age.

In the next chapter you will take the first step in the RENEW program by reducing exposure to toxins in your external environment. Then we will turn to three more actions that you can do to encourage the elimination of toxins from your body and continue to improve your health status. In total, the RENEW program breaks down as follows:

Reduce Eliminate Nourish Energize Wellness

- Reduce (exposure to toxins in your environment)

- Eliminate (current toxins in your body)

- Nourish (your body's cells to support their natural structure, function, and capacity to detoxify)

- Energize (through exercise, physical activity, and relaxation)

- **Wellness.** It helps to keep the "RENEW" acronym in mind every day, because it's not just a program per se. It's a way of life. You will continue to employ the main principles of RENEW in your daily decision-making.

What I love about RENEW is that it doesn't necessarily call for a total change in your lifestyle that will be impossible and impractical to follow. The concepts and underlying lessons of RENEW are doable, and you can take this program to any level you want. You may, for instance, not be ready to complete some of the recommendations suggested, and that's okay. This should not be viewed as an all-or-nothing approach. And you are not about to enter the Zone of Hardship, whereby your life is now filled with restrictions, limitations, and no-nos. You know as well as I that any program with that approach is a setup for failure. As I said earlier and will repeat, start by making just slight shifts in your life. Go at your own pace and be patient with your results.

The more toxic a person is, the longer it may take to experience fully the health benefits this can provide. Moreover, because some toxins take time to literally reach and work their way out of the body, it may take time to see and feel the benefits you want. That said, however, I warn you that you may feel immediate results on some level within just a few days. The body is an incredible machine. No sooner will you begin to tweak your diet and environment than you will marshal the signs of better health. And you will sense a dwindling of symptoms that may have been bothering you for as long as you can remember. I witness this over and over again in my clinics and with people who follow my advice. I'm excited for you in this journey, and you should be, too.

I've designed this five-step program with not only your body in mind, but also your good sense. One of my goals was to create a program that anyone could follow and that's affordable and realistic. Every day it's becoming easier and more economical to live a better life as organic foods flood our regular markets and we no longer have to special-order supplements and vitamins. Often we can find exactly what we're looking for at our local grocery store. There is so much that you can do starting today that costs very little but that can have an enormous impact on your health.

To repeat, your body has an enormous capacity to heal itself, and with my RENEW program you will give your body what it needs to operate on all cylinders—without breaking the bank. People who have been transformed by this program continue to reach out to me and share their success. There is no limit as to what this program can do for you and your health. So let's begin!

Chapter 2 Summary

- Toxins are poisonous substances taken into or produced by the body that can cause illness and disease if allowed to build up over time in the body tissues.

- It's unrealistic to think we can totally eliminate all the toxic substances in the world and their risk factors. The goal is to limit and manage our exposure to them and do what we can to support the natural structures and functions of our bodies so they can detoxify as efficiently as possible.

- Toxins hide out in unlikely places in the body—bones, muscles, fat cells, brain tissue, the liver and other organs—where they can do serious damage, both acutely in the short term and chronically in the long term. Because many fat-soluble toxins park themselves in fat cells, they can mess with signals from these cells that affect our hormones, and that in turn change our metabolism and how we store (or burn) fat.

- RENEW is a comprehensive program to reduce your exposure to toxins in your environment while at the same time flush toxins currently trapped in your body. RENEW follows a straightforward, five-step plan of action:

    Reduce Eliminate Nourish Energize Wellness
    - Reduce (exposure to toxins in your environment)
    - Eliminate (current toxins in your body)
    - Nourish (your body's cells to support their natural structure, function, and capacity to detoxify)
    - Energize (through exercise, physical activity, and relaxation)
    - Wellness.

CHAPTER 3

STEP ONE: REDUCE EXPOSURE TO TOXINS IN YOUR ENVIRONMENT

☙

When actress Kelly Preston took her two-year-old son, Jett, to the hospital in 1994 during a serious health scare in which her boy's immune system seemingly shut down, she later learned that other kids had suffered similar illnesses. Kawasaki syndrome is characterized by high fever, rashes, swollen lymph glands, and pain. Doctors do not understand the syndrome's origin, but when Preston dug a little deeper and examined reports from other families, she noticed that all had cleaned their carpets recently.

☙

No one knew whether Jett would survive. With the help of a medical intervention in which doctors managed to lower his fever and give his immune system a boost through medication, Jett pulled through and slowly recovered. He now lives with allergies. Preston believes his exposure to the residues and the gases coming off the professionally cleaned carpets caused his reaction.

Today Preston is an advocate for chemical-free homes and a staunch supporter of programs that promote a chemical-free world, such as Healthy Children Healthy World (www.healthychild.org). The organization (formerly known as CHEC, or Children's Health Environmental Coalition) boasts an impressive roster of supporters from celebrity and leadership circles who are dedicated to protecting the health and well-being of children from harmful environmental exposures. It was founded by James and Nancy Chuda in 1991 after their daughter Colette died from Wilms' tumor, a rare form of nonhereditary cancer. Unfortunately, children can sometimes bear the brunt of our toxic environment. Their bodies are still developing, especially their immune systems, and they tend to come into greater contact with surfaces and objects that can potentially contain dangerous residues or vapors. A baby crawling on a soft and plush yet chemically treated carpet can pick up more hazards than from a cold, concrete floor.

Six Essential Steps to Reducing Toxins in Your Environment

- Install air filters or commit to proper ventilation
- Buy water filters
- Go room to room and ditch the toxic household goods and products over time, replacing them with all-natural, nontoxic alternatives
- Make your own cleaning products or purchase environmentally friendly ones
- Eat organic whenever possible
- Enhance digestion with enzyme and probiotic supplements

In the United States, the total number of environmentally caused (and preventable) deaths per year was more than twice the amount of deaths due to alcohol consumption, motor vehicle accidents, firearms, and illicit drugs *combined* in 2006. So many of our most prevalent toxins can be found in our building materials, fabrics, furnishings, and gardens. Of course, it's impractical to renovate suddenly or fully remodel our homes and interiors. That cannot be the only solution. But you can do a lot to change the toxic climate by virtue of methodical, step-by-step replacements of materials and sources of chemicals, including cleaning, beauty, and pest control products. This will detoxify your home and put a stop to the level of pollution entering it. It's the R in RENEW: Reduce. By focusing on what you put into your body, as well as the products you buy and the businesses you support, you are taking the first step toward reducing your overall toxic burden and regaining control of your health.

R IS FOR REDUCE

During lectures I usually liken the R: Reduce process to having a broken screen on a window in your house. You have two options: you can continue to clean the house rigorously with no end in sight or you can fix the screen so it no longer lets in all that dirt and dust and bugs. If you keep cleaning the house but never address the source of the problem, you may as well make it your full-time job. What we want to do first and foremost is reduce your current exposure to toxins, then we will clean your biological house. This reduction process will begin to alleviate the toxic strain that your body is enduring and that may be causing underlying problems now or in the future.

Below are specific ideas to consider that will help you achieve a reduction in toxic exposure. Remember, do not feel you must complete all these steps or attempt all the techniques today. Do what you can given your personal needs and resources. The process of detoxification can be done gradually and simply become a habit of your everyday life.

CLEAN UP
YOUR AIR AND WATER

Identifying your top sources of toxins is a natural first step, and for virtually everyone the air and household water is a prime target. This is true whether you live in a major metropolitan area or on a farm, as both locations present problems with air quality; it's nearly impossible to find a place anywhere in the world that has not been affected by pollution. Surprisingly, studies show that your risk of getting cancer from exposure to chemicals in the water and air in your home is actually greater than your risk from exposure to the same chemicals in a hazardous waste site.

Common Sources of Indoor Pollution

aerosol sprays	insulation foam	plastics
asbestos	lawn and garden chemicals	plywood, particleboard
bleach		polyurethane, varnish
carbon monoxide	lead	radon
carpets (synthetic), carpet adhesive	mold	room deodorizers
	mothballs, moth crystals	Styrofoam***
cleaning materials*		synthetic fabrics
dry-cleaned clothing	newsprint	tap water
gasoline	paint, paint remover	tobacco smoke
glue, rubber cement	permanent markers/pens	wood preservatives
heating systems or appliances**	personal care products	
	pesticides	

*Including scouring pads and powders, oven cleaners, detergents, disinfectants, floor and furniture polish and wax, and pot cleaners

**Gas, oil, kerosene, propane, or coal

***Cups, plates, bowls, meat-wrapping materials

Air Purifiers

Volatile organic compounds (VOCs) are mostly to blame for making your indoors so toxic. These are among the same toxins found in new cars, giving them that plasticky (and quintessential) "new car" smell. VOCs, which include chemicals such as acetate, ethanol, and formaldehyde, have been found to have toxic effects, even at low doses. Many are suspected carcinogens. These chemically unstable compounds vaporize (turn to gas) readily and may combine with other chemicals to create compounds that can cause toxic reactions when inhaled or absorbed through the skin. VOCs can be found in cologne and can be released by many other products in your home: carpet adhesives, glues, resins, paints, varnishes, paint strippers and other solvents, wood preservatives, foam insulation, bonding agents, aerosol sprays, cleansers, degreasers and disinfectants, moth repellents, air fresheners, stored fuels, hobby supplies, dry-cleaned clothing, and cosmetics.

TIP

Use plants such as spider plants, aloe vera, chrysanthemum, Gerber daisies, fern, ivy, and philodendrons to help filter toxins from your household air and add oxygen.

Even though you will be doing what you can to reduce these airborne chemicals in the future by choosing eco-friendly alternatives wherever possible, I highly recommend investing in a good air purifier for your home. Airborne chemicals pose one of the greatest pollution threats in the home—and they will pollute you rather easily. There are air purifiers designed for smog, smoke, and particles; for chemicals, gases, and fumes; and for mold, viruses, and bacteria. Some are designed to handle it all. It just depends on what the main indoor concern may be and how much you want to spend. More than 90 percent of particulates you want to filter are small enough to be handled by a HEPA (high efficiency particle absorption) filter. If you suffer from allergies or asthma, air purifiers can help reduce your symptoms. (Try www.air-purifiers-america.com as a start.) Also change the air-conditioning filters in your house often. Get the ducts cleaned yearly.

If you don't want to invest in an air filter today, the simplest and quickest way to keep your air toxins low at home is to be diligent about ventilating your house frequently. Open the windows! Get some cross-ventilation going by opening windows at opposite ends of a room or section of the house. Do this for thirty minutes a day and, if you live near a highway or road, avoid peak traffic hours.

Water Filters

Second, I also recommend buying a household water filter or at least install one on each major faucet. You can do this yourself or hire a professional to come in and install a more sophisticated system. Again, let your budget and personal situation be your guide.

There are a variety of water treatment technologies available today, and it's up to you to decide which one best suits your circumstances and the investment you want to make. Obviously, if you live in an apartment building or co-op, you will be limited as to what you can do, but using individual filters on each faucet can work tremendously well. Some things to consider:

How Bad Is Your Water?

Unfortunately, this question cannot be answered easily based on how your water looks and tastes. Numerous toxins can still be in your water without your sensing it. If you receive your water from a public water supply, you can get a general idea about the quality of your water by researching your community's Annual Quality Report. Check the NRDC report "What's On Tap?" at www.nrdc.org, and ask your water utility (the company that sends you your water bill) for a copy of their annual water quality report. This report will list the detected contaminants, the potential source(s) of those contaminants, and the levels at which those contaminants were present in the water supply.

If you need help reading your report, the NRDC's "Making Sense of 'Right to Know' Reports" can help you decipher it. If you have young kids, are pregnant, or are thinking about pregnancy in the future, you'll want to test your tap water for lead contamination, since lead is especially dangerous and levels can vary enormously from house to house. A lead test costs about $25. Once you know what's in your water, you can find a filter that's geared toward getting rid of the specific pollutants, if any, that may be present.

Don't forget also to consider additional contaminants unique to your home and that may be present in your individual water supply, such as copper, which may be leaching from your household plumbing. If you have a well, you can hire someone to conduct private testing. Local public health departments frequently offer basic water testing services, while private drinking water laboratories can analyze your well water for additional contaminants that are of special concern to residents of your region of the country. Common analyses performed on well water supplies include tests for bacteria (total coliform), nitrates, and hardness. In addition, well water can also be checked for herbicides and pesticides if you live in an agricultural area. You may also choose to have tests performed for radon or arsenic, especially if these contaminants are a common problem in groundwater in your region.

Finding the Right Filter

Filters can be configured in many ways, and they have varying types of mechanical and chemical reduction capabilities. Although some are designed to filter water for the whole house, a majority of the systems on the market today are designed to treat water coming from a single faucet. Some filters must be filled manually, such as a pitcher, while others, such as faucet filters and under-sink systems, are attached directly to the plumbing. Some filters aim to produce clearer, better-tasting water, while others work to remove contaminants that could affect your health. Many filters use more than one kind of filtration technology. Depending on the design and filter media used in the unit, filters are able to reduce many types of contaminants, including chlorine, chlorination by-products, lead, viruses, bacteria, and parasites.

It's pretty easy for a generic filter to catch large contaminants such as dirt particles and bacteria. Viruses are smaller in size and require smaller-holed filters. Pesticides and herbicides are the smallest among prominent contaminants, requiring filters that can catch impurities at the submicron level. The approximate size of bacteria is about 0.5 microns, whereas a pesticide chemical is only 0.001 microns. This means it's imperative that whichever filter you choose, it can handle toxins at the submicron level. Otherwise, contaminants will just pass through.

One rule of thumb is to look for filters labeled as meeting NSF/ANSI Standard 53 that are certified to remove the contaminant(s) of concern in your water. This NSF certification program is not perfect, but it does provide some assurance that at least some claims made by the manufacturer have been verified. NSF-certified filters have been independently tested to show that they can reduce levels of certain pollutants under specified conditions. Those that meet Standard 53 make healthy, clean water a priority rather than just focusing on aesthetic qualities.

For many people, an activated carbon filter bearing NSF Standard 53 certification will do an effective job. But if your water contains perchlorate, for example, a rocket fuel ingredient that's been found in dozens of municipal water supplies throughout the country, a simple countertop filter won't do the job. Following is an explanation of common filters.

Activated carbon filter: Used in countertops, faucet filters, and under-sink units, this filter uses the power of positively charged carbon to attract and absorb impurities. It's what's commonly found in Brita and Pur water filtration systems. It gets rid of bad tastes and odors, including chlorine. Standard 53-certified filters also can substantially reduce many hazardous contaminants, including heavy metals such as copper, lead, and mercury; disinfection by-products; parasites such as *Giardia* and *Cryptosporidium*; pesticides; radon; and volatile organic chemicals.

Cation exchange softener: Used in whole-house and point-of-entry units, this unit softens hard water by removing calcium and magnesium, as well as barium and some other ions that can create health hazards.

Distillers: These boil water and condense the purified steam in a separate chamber. You can find distillers for countertops or ones that can be hooked up to the entire house's points of entry. They can also be combined with carbon filters. Distillers can effectively get rid of heavy metals such as cadmium, chromium, copper, lead, and mercury, as well as arsenic, barium, fluoride, selenium, and sodium. A caveat: there may be significant energy costs associated with using a distillation system, which is why these systems are usually designed to produce enough water for drinking and cooking only.

Reverse osmosis units: These are often combined with a carbon filter or UV disinfection unit (see following page). A semipermeable membrane separates impurities from the water. These systems can produce a significant amount of wastewater, however. Because they produce water very slowly, a pressurized storage tank is usually installed so that water is available to meet the demand for drinking and cooking. A special faucet is installed at the kitchen sink to obtain water from the storage tank.

Ultraviolet disinfection units: These use the power of ultraviolet light to kill bacteria and other microorganisms. Typically found under the sink, they can be combined with a carbon filter and sediment screen. UV units remove bacteria and parasites; class A systems protect against harmful bacteria and viruses, including *Cryptosporidium* and *Giardia*, while class B systems are designed to make nondisease-causing bacteria inactive.

It's important that whichever filter you choose, you maintain it well to assure it continues to perform. As contaminants build up, a filter will become less effective, and it can then start to release harmful bacteria or chemicals back into your filtered water. To keep your filter working properly, follow the manufacturer's maintenance directions. Some filters require only a cartridge change, while others are better maintained by a certified professional. Many filter distributors offer maintenance and service contracts for their products. Before buying any water treatment system, compare not only filter prices, but also operating and maintenance costs for the different units.

Given your particular situation, you may need to install or use more than one of the above technologies to cover the contaminants in your water supply. For example, if you have a problem with bacteria and hard water, you can opt for a UV system and a water softener. If arsenic and chlorination by-products are present, you could treat your water with a combination of reverse osmosis and carbon filtration. Don't forget to consider filtration units for showerheads as well. You can find these at major hardware and home improvement stores, as well as specialty stores for kitchens and baths. This will help reduce your exposure to contaminants in the water that can vaporize in the hot, steamy air that you then breathe into your lungs or absorb through your skin. Your skin is your largest organ, and it can also be a welcome mat for toxins that get readily absorbed.

When choosing a specific make and model of a product or system, it is important to know that it is made from materials that are safe for water contact, that it is structurally sound, and that it will perform as claimed by the manufacturer. Many manufacturers will have their products performance tested and certified by an independent organization (e.g., NSF International) to provide some assurance that the product meets standard requirements.

NSF International in particular is one to look for on product labels. NSF is a nonprofit, nongovernmental organization that provides product testing services and risk management solutions to the public. (For further information on drinking water issues, including treatment options, you can contact the NSF Consumer Affairs Office toll-free at 1-877-867-3435 or via e-mail at info@nsf.org.)

A WORD ABOUT MOLD

Mold Reactions

respiratory problems, such as wheezing and difficulty breathing

nasal and sinus congestion

burning, watery, red eyes; blurred vision; light sensitivity

dry, hacking cough

sore throat

nose and throat irritation

shortness of breath

skin irritation

central nervous system problems (constant headaches, memory problems, and mood changes)

aches and pains

possible fever

Mold simply refers to fungal growth. If you had a mold problem in your home or office, you'd know it, right? Not necessarily. The sobering fact is that mold can grow and multiply in concealed areas of a building—in air ducts, attics, and wall cavities—without producing obvious signs, but taking a toll upon your health nonetheless.

Fungi require moisture to grow, and most reproduce by releasing spores. Mold growth can be arrested by removing and replacing water-damaged building materials, cleaning exposed surfaces, and controlling indoor humidity. However, if moldy materials are not properly removed (by professionals under "containment" conditions) and all affected surfaces thoroughly cleaned, other areas of the building may become contaminated with mold spores, spreading the problem. And even if spores are no longer alive, allergens and mycotoxins could still be present that may affect your health."

There is growing recognition today of the serious health threat that mold poses, as well as how problematic—and costly—its identification and remediation can be. For this reason, some have dubbed mold "the new asbestos."

While allergic reaction to mold (experienced by one in three people) is the most common health problem associated with exposure, many symptoms (either alone or in combination) may also result.

If you suspect that mold is a problem in your home, I encourage you to hire a certified inspector who specializes in detecting this biological toxin. Many of these inspectors are not the same people who do remediation, which is the proper procedure for removal and cleanup. You can get a fair evaluation of your situation and consider your options for taking care of any mold or mildew that may be present.

CHOOSE NATURAL PRODUCTS TO FILL YOUR HOME AND PERSONAL HYGIENE KITS

The reason for the dramatic increase in our exposure to indoor pollutants is largely due to the construction of more tightly sealed, energy-efficient buildings. These buildings are often poorly ventilated and constructed and furnished with synthetic materials. The escalating use of chemical-based consumer products inside such homes can be a recipe for disaster, especially in consideration of the fact that the average person spends upwards of 90 percent of his time indoors. Chemical contaminants in buildings contribute to "sick building syndrome," which is in reality "sick *person* syndrome," a result of time spent in contaminated buildings. Such exposure can give rise to environmental illness, a growing problem today estimated to affect 40 million Americans (and an area of specialization for some progressive physicians).

We tend to have some idea that the products under the sink—like the stinky sprays, disinfectants, and bleaches—are quite hazardous, but we forget about all the other potential toxins in our daily routines. (And some of us may *not* realize the level of toxicity emanating from our cabinets, as we take for granted cleaning products we falsely think are "safe" and use them liberally around the house, and around our families and children.)

When the National Institute for Occupational Safety and Health (NIOSH) analyzed 2,983 chemicals used in personal care products, they found that 884 of the chemicals were toxic, 314 caused biological mutations, 218 caused reproductive complications, and 778 caused acute toxicity. The average adult uses about nine personal care products a day, totaling about 126 chemicals. At least one-third of the ingredients used in these products have been noted to cause cancer or some other serious health problem. Industrial chemicals are basic ingredients in personal care products and 89 percent of 10,500 ingredients used in these products have not been evaluated for safety.

Among the most damaging personal care products are those that are scented, including cologne, deodorants, lotions, creams, bath salts, shampoo, cosmetics, soaps, body powders, and oils. Scented products can contain up to 5,000 different chemicals in various combinations, the vast majority of which have had little or no human toxicology testing.

Cosmetics contain not only fragrances (with all their component chemicals) but also metal salts. Mascara and eyeliners may contain lead or coal tar dyes, which are also found in hair dyes. In addition, hair dyes contain aniline dyes, known to cause cancer in animals. Body powders made with talc can cause scarring of lung tissue when fine particles are inhaled. Some shampoos and hair conditioners, hand lotions, and hair colors contain a potentially dangerous antibacterial chemical called methylisothiazolinone (MIT).

The good news in this is that you can make the most improvements in your life through minimal changes. It's pretty easy to swap out your old products for natural, environmentally friendly ones that can do the same job. It's also important to read labels, even though all ingredients are not always listed. If those that are listed are unknown to you and difficult to pronounce, chances are they are potentially toxic chemicals that are best avoided.

Cleaning products may lie at the top of the list for concentrations of toxicity in your home, but if you don't use them every day, then it may be more relevant to start looking in your bathroom, bedroom, main rooms, and home office first. We assume the products we purchase at our local department or home improvement store have all been safety-tested and have a seal of approval for home usage. But, as we have seen, they can all be toxic. And aside from what we fill our cupboards and cabinets with, up to 80 percent of the materials used in today's indoor environments are artificial. Such materials release dangerous chemicals that are then inhaled. (Reminder: Refer to Chapter 9 for a complete "day in the life" tour of our toxin-filled homes and daily habits.)

Bathroom and Vanity

Take a good look in your main bathroom, where you probably spend several minutes each day getting ready for the day or bed. Take everything out of the cabinets, drawers, and cosmetic bags, and get rid of the old outdated stuff you think you might use one day but haven't for five years now! Look at the ingredients in your toothpaste, shampoo, conditioner, soap, hair spray, and so on. Choose one or two products a week to replace with a natural product that does not contain the harsh toxic chemicals.

An increasing number of companies are beginning to sell products that lack potential or known toxins. Natural beauty and personal care products made without added chemicals or unnecessary ingredients can usually be found in most health food stores. I'm a huge fan of Aubrey Organics, which sells a great line of all natural shampoos, conditioners, body lotions, makeup, and even baby and pet products. By using natural preservatives such as vitamin E and grapefruit seed extract, they avoid the addition of chemical preservatives. The following are the top ten synthetic cosmetic ingredients to avoid. Aubrey Hampton calls them the "10 most wanted"; I recommend visiting the site at www.aubrey-organics.com for more information.

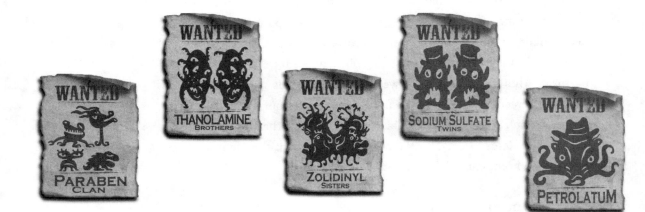

TOXINS: THE **10** MOST WANTED LIST

Methyl, propyl, butyl, and ethyl paraben: These villains help extend the shelf life of products and prevent microbial growth. But not only can they trigger allergic reactions and skin rashes, studies have shown that they are weakly estrogenic and can be absorbed by the body through the skin. Parabens could be responsible for accelerating the growth of tumors in the breast. Because parabens are used in commercial deodorants, particularly antiperspirants, scientists are now considering a link between the use of common deodorants and an increased risk of breast cancer in women. A woman is eight times more likely to develop breast cancer in the area of the breast closest to the underarm than in any other part of the breast.

Diethanolamine (DEA), triethanolamine (TEA): As emulsifiers and/or foaming agents, these villains also can cause allergic reactions, eye irritations, and dryness of hair and skin. Both of these chemicals are ammonia compounds, which means they can combine with nitrates to form carcinogenic compounds called nitrosamines.

Diazolidinyl urea, imidazolidinyl urea: These widely used preservatives are blamed for contact dermatitis. Two trade names for these chemicals are Germall II and Germall 115. Both release formaldehyde, which as you know can be toxic.

Sodium lauryl/laureth sulfate: This is a cheap, harsh detergent used in shampoos for its cleansing and foam-building properties. Often derived from petroleum, it is frequently disguised in pseudo-natural cosmetics with the phrase "comes from coconuts." It causes eye irritation, scalp scurf similar to dandruff, skin rashes, and other allergic reactions.

Petrolatum: Also known as petroleum jelly, this mineral oil derivative is used for its emollient properties in cosmetics. It has no nutrient value for the skin and can interfere with the body's own natural moisturizing mechanism, leading to dryness and chapping. It often creates the very conditions it claims to alleviate. Manufacturers use petrolatum because it is unbelievably cheap.

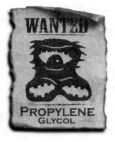

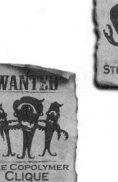

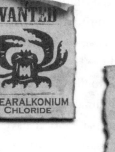

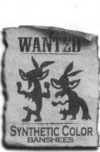

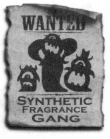

Propylene glycol: Ideally this is a vegetable glycerin mixed with grain alcohol, both of which are natural. Usually it is a synthetic petrochemical mix used as a humectant. It has been known to cause allergic reactions, hives, and eczema. When you see PEG (polyethylene glycol) or PPG (polypropylene glycol) on labels, take note—these are related synthetics.

PVP/VA copolymer: This is a petroleum-derived chemical used in hair sprays, styling aids, and other cosmetics. It can be considered toxic, since inhaled particles can be damaging to the lungs of sensitive people.

Stearalkonium chloride: This is an ammonium compound used in hair conditioners and creams that may cause allergic reactions. It was developed by the fabric industry as a fabric softener and is a lot cheaper and easier to use in hair conditioning formulas than proteins or herbals, which are beneficial to the hair.

Synthetic colors: Synthetic colors, along with synthetic hair dyes, should be avoided at all costs. They will be labeled as FD&C or D&C, followed by a color and a number. Example: FD&C Red No. 6 / D&C Green No. 6. Many synthetic colors can be carcinogenic. If a cosmetic contains them, don't use it.

Synthetic fragrances: The synthetic fragrances used in cosmetics can have hundreds of ingredients. There is no way to know what the chemicals are, since on the label it will simply read "fragrance." Some problems caused by these chemicals include headaches, dizziness, rash, hyperpigmentation, violent coughing, vomiting, skin irritation—the list goes on. Try to avoid buying a cosmetic that has the word "fragrance" on the ingredients label.

Surprisingly, cosmetics ingredients don't fall under the jurisdiction of either the EPA or the Food and Drug Administration, and many such products sold in the United States today contain known toxins. Formaldehyde and toluene, both identified by the EPA as carcinogens, are part of the mix in many common cosmetics, including nail care products, as are phthalates, chemicals that have been linked to birth defects. Cosmetics manufacturers are now required to disclose dangerous ingredients to the State Department of Health and Human Services, but they are not required to remove them. For a list of companies that have pledged to not use harmful chemicals, visit http://www.safecosmetics.org. For ideas on natural skin care, see the recipes that follow.

Natural Skin Care Recipes

Citrus Sugar Scrub

2 cups	white cane sugar
2 cups	vegetable glycerin
1 teaspoon	vitamin C crystals
5 drops	orange essential oil

Combine ingredients in a bowl. Scoop some scrub onto your hand and massage gently over entire body. Rinse well with warm water. Store remainder in a glass jar. Keep in a cool, dry place and use within two weeks.

Lavender Salt Glow

2 cups	fine sea salt
4 cups	almond oil
30 drops	lavender essential oil

Place all ingredients in a wide-mouth jar. Mix together. To use, wet entire body and massage onto skin. Rinse well and towel off to dry.

If it's too overwhelming to replace all your bathroom goods at once, aim to replace one or two products a week with natural ones. Keep in mind that "unscented" does not mean a product contains no fragrance. Ingredients used to mask unpleasant odors, usually chemicals, do not have to be identified on the labels. "Hypoallergenic" can also be misleading. This term applies to *known* allergens. A product that is hypoallergenic may still contain ingredients that irritate you or that have not yet been listed as possible "allergens."

Nontoxic Deodorants and Soaps

The most active ingredient in most deodorants is aluminum chlorohydrate, a known toxin that can be readily absorbed through the skin. There are plenty of alternative products that can naturally deodorize sweat and, coupled with good hygiene, will provide you with more than adequate protection. Tom's of Maine, for example, can be found at most health food stores and offers an array of hygiene products, including a line of natural deodorants and toothpastes.

Expunge the antibacterial soaps. I know they've been enormously popular recently but they will kill the good bacteria along with the bad. They may also contribute to the development of antibiotic-resistant strains of bacteria. All-natural soaps will do the job without robbing you of the bacteria you need to maintain good health and a robust immune system.

A Chemical-Free Bedroom

Next, consider your bedding, closets, and clothing. We spend about a third of our time in the bedroom (and, above all, in bed) so it's wise to make this spot as chemical free as possible. Start replacing your old sheets with organic cotton sheets (check out a company called Gaiam at www.gaiam .com). There are many companies that offer bedding products made without toxic flame-retardant chemicals, using naturally flame-retardant fibers instead. Hästens is one such company, but they may be too expensive for some. You can start by purchasing a natural mattress cover that fits snugly over your current mattress and that will help prevent the off-gassing from passing through. Use hypoallergenic pillows filled with natural fibers like cotton, wool, and feathers.

To insulate yourself from the sea of synthetics in your bed:

- Use a hypoallergenic mattress cover or an extra layer of blankets and sheets made of 100 percent natural fibers such as cotton or wool.

- Consider a whole new, hypoallergenic bed or top mattress like the one made by Hästens (www.hastens.com/en-us/accessories/top-mattresses).

- Use pillows filled with natural fibers.

- Sleep in natural clothes made of fabrics that have not been chemically treated (i.e., avoid fabrics labeled "permanent press," "wrinkle resistant," "antistatic," and "water or stain repellent").

Reduce the electrical devices and cords in your bedroom by keeping them out or at least away from the bed. They generate electric and magnetic fields that may or may not have a negative effect on health. This includes televisions, computers, and radios (you'll sleep better with these distracting objects out!). Use a battery-operated clock.

Take inventory of your closet and clear out clothes made of unnatural fibers. Make a mental note to avoid buying clothes that require dry cleaning. Choose natural fibers such as cotton, linen, wool, and hemp. When you do choose to dry-clean certain pieces, let them aerate *outside* for a day before placing them in your closet or wearing them. (And be sure to remove any plastic covering from the cleaners!)

A Room with a Fume

Carpets, fabrics, and upholstery are prime spots for toxins, due to the flame retardants and solvents. Make it a goal to think about replacing these over time with products that are not made with chemicals. I recommend starting with flooring because carpeting in particular is a magnet for dust and toxic chemicals roaming elsewhere in the household and that land on the floor eventually. This includes household pesticide residues and cleaning agents—even if they were not originally applied to the carpet.

When reflooring, consider natural-fiber carpeting that is manufactured without additives and that does not have the formaldehyde and other chemicals (examples include wool, hemp, cotton, or jute). Organic carpeting is getting easier to find. A better choice for flooring would be ceramic tile, wood, or other noncarpet materials free of most of the chemicals found in carpeting and carpet cleaners. Washable throw rugs are also a good choice, and can be easier to clean.

The following "recipes" give you ideas on natural cleaning mixes and products that will help you clean your floors and carpets toxin-free. Old-fashioned baking soda works like magic as a carpet deodorizer. White vinegar and water is an excellent stain remover and general carpet cleaner. For a heavy-duty job, you can steam-clean your carpets every few months or as needed. When you are ready to buy your next vacuum, choose one that has a HEPA filter, and vacuum at least twice a week.

Natural Household Cleaning Product Recipes

All-Purpose Window Wash

¼ cup	white distilled vinegar
½ teaspoon	liquid soap or detergent
2 cups	water

Combine all ingredients in a spray bottle and shake to blend. Spray, then remove with a paper towel or newspaper. Store in a cool, dry place.

Carpet Freshener

4 cups	baking soda
35 drops	eucalyptus essential oil
30 drops	lavender essential oil
25 drops	rosewood essential oil

Mix essential oils and baking soda in a bowl. Break up any clumps that may form, stir until mixed well. Sprinkle powder onto floor and let sit for about 15 minutes, then vacuum. Store in a glass jar, and keep in a cool, dry place.

Lavender All-Purpose Glass Cleaner

¼ cup	white distilled vinegar
½ teaspoon	liquid soap or detergent
2 cups	water
25 drops	pure lavender antiseptic essential oil

Combine all ingredients in a spray bottle and shake to blend. Spray, and then wipe area with a paper towel or newspaper.

Lavender Soft Scrubber

½ cup	baking soda
1 cup	liquid soap or detergent
10 drops	pure lavender antiseptic essential oil

Place baking soda in a bowl. Slowly mix in liquid soap (enough to make a frosting-like consistency—this will depend on the hardness of your water), stirring constantly until it is the consistency of frosting. Add lavender oil. Place the mix directly onto a sponge and use.

Note: This will start to harden rather quickly, so make only what you need. You may also add some pure vegetable glycerin to the baking soda mix so it will stay softer longer. Just place unused scrubber in a jar and seal the lid tightly. You will find all-purpose liquid detergents and all-purpose soaps at most health food stores.

Lemon Floor Wash

¼ cup	liquid soap or detergent
½ cup	lemon juice
½ cup	white distilled vinegar
25 drops	lemon essential oil
1 gallon	water

Combine all ingredients in a bucket. Mix until soapy. Mop or sponge to clean the floor as normal, and rinse.

Lemon Furniture Polish

| 1 cup | olive oil |
| ½ cup | lemon juice |

Combine ingredients in a spray bottle and shake well to mix. Apply a small amount to a flannel cloth or cleaning rag. Spread evenly over surface. Turn cloth to other side and polish dry.

Paint can pose serious health risks. If you know you have lead paint on your walls or woodwork (i.e., if you live in a home that was built before 1978), you may want to have a specialist test for lead dust in your carpet. Depending on how bad it is, you can choose to have your carpets cleaned by someone who specializes in removing this kind of dust, or you can put that on your list of things to replace entirely when your budget allows.

There are paints that are available even at local paint stores that produce very few vapors and do not contain the toxic volatile compound usually released from traditional paints. A great place to start looking is www.healthyhomes.com.

Eco-Friendly Garden and Pest Control

Plenty of natural alternatives are now available for garden and pest control in your yard. These will be free of pesticides, herbicides, and fungicides but equally as effective as those that do contain these toxins. They often use ingredients such as diatomaceous earth (made from calcareous fossils) herbs, and oils, such as orange oil or mint oil, that are natural insect repellents. Natural pest control services are also available if you have a large garden to control and you don't want to do this yourself. If you have a gardener, speak with him or her about alternatives to commercial products loaded with toxins or find a new gardener who uses nontoxic products.

If you live near utility poles or any wood that's been treated with pressurized CCA (this chemical, whose full name is chromated copper arsenate, is commonly used to treat wood in decking, garden furniture, and fencing so it can withstand the elements, insects, and fungi), plant a fern close to it. The fern will absorb the arsenic coming off the wood. Because CCA-treated wood can be found in public parks, playgrounds, and perhaps in your own backyard, it would be a good idea to wipe your feet on a doormat before going indoors, and wash your hands. Woods in general tend to be treated with an array of chemicals. If you are uncertain about your own backyard's equipment, you can seal any wood with paint or a polyurethane coating to trap emissions.

Indoor pests can also be taken care of through natural alternatives to toxic bug sprays. Ants can be taken care of by mixing 1 cup water with 2 teaspoons of essential peppermint oil. Spray the mixture where ants are getting in (windowsills, floorboards) and watch them disappear. Baking soda and powdered sugar can send cockroaches packing; and an herbal spray or natural flea collar can help repel fleas on your pet. You can find natural, oil- and plant-based products to use on your pets that will keep them flea free. The best advice of all, however, for keeping your home pest free is to keep it clean and deodorized from the start. Avoid commercial deodorizers, however, and opt instead for natural ones made with essential oils (essential oils are compounds found within aromatic plants). Try citrus oils in your kitchen and flower oils in your bathrooms.

The Lion's Den

Wherever you store household cleaners, detergents, disinfectants, bleaches, stain removers for the laundry, and so on, aim to tackle this place gradually. Replace one or two products a week with natural ones, and try making your own where possible using the ideas on pages 63-65. Every year, about half a million tons of liquid cleaners go down the drain in the United States alone. Household cleaners, which are sold now in virtually all retail outlets, from grocery stores to convenience markets and pharmacies, are the major source of home toxins; they are a toxic cocktail of petroleum-based surfactants, solvents, and other chemicals that are associated with a bevy of health problems. (An exploration of their labeling gives you a clue.) The number one cause of household poisoning is dish detergent.

Any daytime television show will be interrupted with copious commercials touting the amazing cleaning capabilities of this or that. But you don't need anything more than a few basic ingredients to get the job done. As mentioned above, those include water, white vinegar, baking soda, lemon juice, and maybe some borax and hydrogen peroxide. And if do-it-yourself cleaning products aren't for you, there are many brands on the market that do not contain harsh chemicals but work expertly well. Nontoxic, environmentally friendly household cleaners are now available in most health food stores as well as many mass market stores (see Resource Directory, page 265, for leads). These can still be a little pricier than regular toxic cleaners, but your health is worth it. If you feel the need to keep a few regular, chemical-laden cleaning products, store them in airtight containers and keep them in the toolshed or garage.

Home Office

If you have a home office or room where you store arts and crafts, you may want to rethink how you store glues, ink cartridges, liquid paper, rubber cement, carbon paper, and so on. Keep all of these products, which will be labeled as toxic, in sealed containers. As with any other room, you should keep this one well ventilated and place a large plant or two in a corner.

Light It Up Naturally

For all your house's rooms, try to bring in as much natural light as possible so you don't have to resort to so much artificial lighting. Both fluorescent and incandescent lighting lack the full spectrum of wavelengths that exist in sunlight. Depriving yourself of natural sunlight has known health consequences, from chaotic circadian rhythms to depression. Circadian rhythms are the patterns of repeated activity associated with cycles of day and night. Our internal rhythms repeat roughly every twenty-four hours, and involve the sleep-wake cycle, the ebb and flow of hormones, the rise and fall of body temperature, and other subtle rhythms that mesh with the twenty-four-hour solar day.

Spending time each day outside in the natural light is the key to keeping your body's rhythms aligned (it will also get you out of the more polluted indoors). You can also consider installing full-spectrum lighting in places where you spend the most time in your home. These lights can be purchased at home improvement and hardware stores.

EAT ORGANIC WHENEVER POSSIBLE

"Organically grown" food is grown and processed using no synthetic fertilizers or pesticides. But this doesn't mean that "organic" equates with "100 pure" as we'd like to think. Pesticides derived from natural sources (e.g., biological pesticides) may be used in producing organically grown food. And there have been many cases of foods labeled "organic" that test positive for pesticide residues. Reasons for this are pretty logical: soils used to grow organic foods may have been exposed to pesticides in the past that loiter in the ground; and nearby "conventional farming" plots (i.e., lands that use pesticides) share their pesticides when the winds blow. Of course, there's always the mislabeling explanation. A worker packaging lettuce for shipping may accidentally label a box "organic" when in fact it came from the side of the farm that liberally sprays pesticides.

That said, organic foods routinely test higher on the nutrient scale as compared to their conventionally grown counterparts. And when they do carry signs of pesticide exposure, for the most part they contain a far lower amount of chemical residues.

The Detox Diet outlined in Chapter 6, plus the recipes in Chapter 11, will give you greater specifics on how to eat as chemically free as possible and nourish your body with nutrients that will boost your health and enhance your natural detoxification systems. But now is a good time to get ready for that part of the program by thinking about buying organic and taking an honest look at what you have in your kitchen cabinets and refrigerator that could be sabotaging your health and vitality (and even your attempts to lose weight). Eating organic foods offers two benefits: it will help you to reduce your toxin intake, and because organic foods tend to score higher on the nutrient meter, they will support the health of your body's biomechanics and innate detoxification capacity. It's a win-win with organic foods.

The importance of eating organic is gaining momentum. As demand rises, the pricing of organic foods is coming down now into the affordable range. If you have the convenience of a health food store with a good produce section near you, utilize it. But even mass market food stores are now offering a pretty impressive line of organic produce, meats, and other food items. Eat organic fruits and vegetables whenever possible to avoid the chemicals, pesticides, and herbicides generally found in produce. When you do buy conventionally grown produce, peel away the outer skin first. For produce you can't peel, like broccoli, boiling or cooking it will take care of removing most chemicals, but don't forget to discard the water. Choose organic meats and dairy to avoid the hormones and antibiotics. Opt for wild-caught fish and cut down on albacore ("white") tuna and swordfish. Select unprocessed foods to avoid the preservatives, dyes, nitrates, and nitrites.

Going organic will also help you to limit your consumption of processed and refined foods—most of which are packed with excess sodium, unhealthy fats, and sugar. You will also reap the benefits of the natural chemicals that plants have originally made for their own protection. In their own survival efforts, plants use phytonutrients to protect themselves from disease and to boost their own immunity. That's one reason researchers believe organic fruits and vegetables are healthier—they are raised without pesticides, forcing them to produce more of their own protective chemicals.

TIP

Switch from processed peanut butter to raw almond butter or organic peanut butter. Most commercially manufactured nut butters add sugar, oils, preservatives, and other additives to the mix. Read the ingredients and make sure you don't see anything but 100 percent nuts. Keep organic fresh fruit and veggies cut up in the fridge, and make smoothies using fresh fruits such as bananas, berries, and orange juice.

Detoxify Your Kitchen

I recommend cleaning out your kitchen and throwing away foods containing suspicious ingredients—coloring agents, chemical additives, and preservatives (you'll know them when you can't pronounce them). Get rid of the Hamburger Helper. Besides being full of unnecessary and unhealthy ingredients, these types of foods add no nutritional value. Usually the fewer ingredients the better. It is better to get real butter than margarine, better to get real sugar than artificial sweeteners, and so on. Just use them in moderation.

Avoid These

high-fructose corn syrup

hydrogenated and partially hydrogenated oils

enriched and bleached flour

artificial sweeteners (aspartame, saccharine, sucralose, acesulfame potassium, and cyclamate potassium)

monosodium glutamate (MSG)

modified cornstarch

sugar

bromate

olestra (brand name Olean)

colorings known as FD&C Red No. 3, Yellow No. 6, Blue No. 1, Blue No. 2, and Green No. 3

If there is something that you feel you just can't live without, then save it and eat it once in a while—moderation! Try the 80/20 rule. Eighty percent of the time eat foods that you know are going to nourish your body: fresh fruit, veggies, lean proteins, wild fish, raw nuts, seeds, yogurt, and salads. Then once in a while treat yourself with something that you know is not on your list of good things. I say this because you have to make the lifestyle doable!

Try shopping the perimeter of a grocery store, as this is where the fresh produce, meats, and dairy will be. You will be avoiding most of the processed and refined products that are generally located in interior aisles of grocery stores. Watch out for prepackaged food products tucked in the perimeter and screaming "simple and easy." Most packaged food items, especially those targeted toward our children, are filled with preservatives, chemical additives, and coloring agents which research has shown contribute to attention deficit problems.

The recipes starting on page 241 will show you how to sauté your vegetables with water instead of resorting to high-fat, low-quality oils. When you do use an oil, try to use extra virgin olive oil or canola oil. Nuts, seeds, and avocados are all excellent sources of healthy oils, but you'll want to consume them in moderation due to their high fat content. Select raw, organic nuts and seeds (such as pumpkin, sesame, and sunflower) whenever possible, and soak them overnight to deactivate enzyme inhibitors and thus improve their digestibility.

Stock Up on Organic Herbs and Spices

When it comes to condiments and spices, we often resort to items that are full of preservatives, additives, and refined sugars. I challenge you to explore your pantry or the door to your refrigerator and see just how many odd-sounding ingredients you find on bottles, jars, and shakers. For example, regular ketchup and BBQ sauce can be loaded with additives, especially high-fructose corn syrup.

You can do so much better with just natural, organic spices and herbs. Organic sauces and condiments can also be found in many stores today.

Healthy Seasonings

lemon and lemon juice

light soy sauce

balsamic vinegar

mustard

chilies

pepper

garlic

coarse salt

Worcestershire sauce

Beware of Genetically Modified Foods

Genetically modified (GM) foods are foods produced from organisms that have had a part of their genetic makeup—their DNA—altered through genetic engineering. Many scientists and politicians believe that making plants resistant to insects and infections will greatly increase crop yield and help prevent world hunger. In fact, in 2006 a total of 252 million acres of transgenic (or GM) crops were planted in twenty-two countries by 10.3 million farmers. The United States led the way with 53 percent of its crops produced from GM organisms, followed by Argentina (17 percent), Brazil (11 percent), Canada (6 percent), India (4 percent), and China (3 percent). The majority of these crops were herbicide- and insect-resistant soybeans, corn, cotton, canola, and alfalfa.

Another use of this technology is to produce a GM rice with increased iron and vitamins, which could alleviate chronic malnutrition in third-world countries. So on the surface it looks like this technology would be helpful to humans. Unfortunately, there is more data showing up to suggest there could be serious negative side effects using GM foods. It's important to note that we don't have a requirement in the United States to label foods as genetically modified if they in fact have come from this technology. What's more, estimates suggest that 80 percent of the soy production in the United States is genetically modified and over half of the corn planted in the country has been genetically modified (which, by the way, contributes to the production of copious amounts of high-fructose corn syrup among other products). The jury is still out on what this could mean for human health and the environment. Apparently the only way you can be certain you are not eating a GM food is to eat only organic food, which is a great idea in any case.

Switch to Nontoxic Cooking and Storage Wares

Avoid plastics, nonstick wares, and aluminums when you store (and for that matter, cook) foods. Use nonplastic wares, containers, and wrappings, such as ceramics, porcelain, glass, and natural parchment paper.

ENHANCE DIGESTION WITH ENZYMES AND PROBIOTICS

Up to now, I've been covering mostly external toxins. But remember that there are two types of toxins—those that originate from your outside environment and those that arise from your body's normal functions. Everyday physiological processes such as energy production, digestion, and hormone synthesis create waste products that, if not discarded, interfere with the function of your internal organs. Internal toxicity is the process by which the body produces toxic substances that are self-destructive. As humans we perform only two broad physiological functions. First, we take in and absorb nutrients, and second, we expel waste and toxins. We excrete these toxins mostly when we urinate (in urine) or eliminate (in fecal matter), but also to a lesser degree when we breathe, sweat, cut our hair, and trim our nails.

Most of these wastes are the by-products of the air we breathe and the food we eat. However, our intestinal tracts are full of bacteria and yeasts that also produce waste. These bacteria and yeasts are often called gut flora or intestinal microbes. Some of these bacteria are highly beneficial. They assist with the digestion of some vitamins and they play a significant roll in our immune response. About 100 trillion (three pounds) of these bacteria live in the intestinal tracts of virtually every human on earth. In fact, we have more of these microbes living in our intestinal tract than we have cells in our body (only about 80 trillion). These bacteria are either good for you, bad for you, or neutral.

When people ask me about the number one root cause of most chronic illness, they are often surprised when I say poor digestion and an inability to detoxify efficiently is likely to blame. They are also amazed to learn that the body itself can produce harmful toxins; it's counterintuitive to think that the human body is able to create and harbor structures and substances that can lead to its self-destruction. But it can. And it will if you present the right conditions.

Although environmental toxins are most certainly an important contributing factor, digestive toxins, which include those produced by harmful microbes in our gastrointestinal tracts, are an equally important, though often overlooked, source of disease in the body. Combined, both external and internal toxins are a double whammy. They make for a heavier body burden as well as a dysfunctional digestive system, which can contribute to all manner of disease, not just gastrointestinal disorders.

When properly digested, carbohydrates are converted to glucose, protein to amino acids, and fats are broken down into glycerin and fatty acids. If these conversions are incomplete, food will not be in the proper form for our bodies to absorb. That food will therefore pass through the system undigested (or partially digested), producing toxins as a result. If the body is unable to promptly eliminate these toxins, either because the toxic load is too great or because detoxification channels (specific organs and systems discussed in the next chapter) are blocked (or both), they will be retained and lead ultimately to disease.

If you suffer chronic digestive problems such as constipation, irritable bowel syndrome, and gastrointestinal reflux disease (GERD), you would do well to consider supplementing your diet with digestive enzymes at each meal. These will help you further digest your food better and reduce the production of digestive by-products that can lead to intestinal toxicity. You'll learn more about digestive enzymes in Chapter 6. They serve two duties: they help keep your digestive tract running smoothly so you limit your exposure to intestinal toxins, and because they enhance digestion they will also support your entire detoxification system.

In addition, a good probiotic supplement will also assist with keeping the intestinal ecology in the proper balance. Friendly intestinal bacteria (also known as flora or probiotics, which literally means "for life"), can help your body destroy bad bacteria and keep a fine balance in your digestive tract that will further help you absorb the nutrients you need so your natural detoxification systems continue to run smoothly. Again, I'll be giving you more direction about probiotics in Chapter 6. For now, understand that the addition of supplemental probiotics and digestive enzymes are part of your overall strategy for removing toxins and reducing your exposure to them.

Chapter 3 Summary

Step One : Reduce Exposure to Toxins in Your Environment

You do this through:

- Cleaning up your air and water
- Choosing natural products in your home
- Creating chemical-free rooms in your home
- Eating organic whenever possible
- Enhancing digestion with enzymes and probiotics

THE BEAUTY OF YOUR BODY'S NATURAL DETOX METHODS

❧

Evolution has made sure that our bodies can defend themselves against harmful encounters. On the most elementary level, when you reflexively pull your hand away from a hot stove, this is a normal response programmed by your body's internal mechanics. When you catch a cold or get an infection, your immune system kicks into overdrive to kill the invading virus or bacteria. And when you consume a food laced with non-nutrients—from caffeine to synthetic chemicals—your liver is one of the many channels that help process and clean out elements your body cannot use for life-sustaining energy.

❧

But there are lots of reasons to be concerned that our bodies cannot fulfill this role 100 percent of the time for all the things to which we expose it. We simply have not evolved fast enough to keep up with the surge in toxins we've released into the world. I think it's quite telling that the

Centers for Disease Control and Prevention admit that as much as 80 percent of all illnesses have environmental and lifestyle causes. The bright silver lining: this tips the scales—putting the power of health and wellness into our hands. If the odds of getting sick are based mostly on how we choose to live, from what we eat to the air we breathe and how we take care of our bodies, then we can choose to live healthily. We can choose to avoid illness. All too often, we may feel as if illness happens to us. Now it's time to see a different side to this picture.

Let's focus on how we can make our lifestyles better and our bodies more robust. In doing so, we will also begin to effect changes in our toxic world. As we work toward cleaning out our bodies, homes, and living spaces, each of us will be doing our small part in cleaning out the world on a global scale. At the same time we will be encouraging industries, societies, and governments to make changes that will also contribute to the massive cleanup.

As I've noted, toxins can be a variety of factors we come into contact with every day of our lives. They include heavy metals and a range of chemicals such as pesticides, pollutants, and food additives that have become almost unavoidable—an inevitable price to pay for the advancements we have made as a human race. With the yin of progress comes the yang of consequence. We have created some toxins that are so foreign to our bodies that they just don't know what to do with them, so instead of effectively neutralizing or eliminating them, these toxins get thrown into remote corners of tissues and organs, and especially fat cells, where they can sit for years and cause irreparable damage. Drugs, tobacco, and alcohol also have toxic effects in the body even when they originate from wholly natural sources. And then there are those toxins that get produced as normal by-products of digestion, including intestinal bacteria that break down food.

Now that you have learned how to create a safer and healthier home, it's time to reduce your body's internal toxic load and nourish yourself with the biological tools necessary for supporting a vigorous human body. A vigorous human body is one that can effectively detoxify—combat incoming toxins while flushing out processed toxins—and whose cellular units are fully functional so they can do their specific job, whatever that may be. You have cells that allow your heart to beat, your brain to think, your immune system to fight disease and injury, your body to move, your eyes to see, your fingers to feel, and so on and so forth. Detoxification is an important function that goes on every second in every cell, and it's arguably the body's central generator for your overall wellness.

Because it helps to have an understanding of how detoxification happens within the body automatically (i.e., without you really thinking about it), we're going to start here in this chapter with an overview of the body's main channels of detoxification. Then we'll return to the steps in the RENEW program.

THE BODY'S DETOX METHODS

In Deepak Chopra's *Magical Mind, Magical Body: Mastering the Mind/Body Connection for Perfect Health and Total Well-Being*, the author points out some amazing facts about our body's capacity to heal itself. Quantum physicists have proven that 98 percent of the atoms in your body are replaced within one year. In three months your body produces an entirely new skeleton. Every six weeks, all the cells have been replaced in your liver. You have a new stomach lining every five days. You are continually replacing old blood cells with new ones. Your skin is sloughing off dead cells and producing a new skin monthly. The proteins in your muscles are in a constant state of flux as amino acids are catabolized (broken down into smaller units and released as energy) and new muscle tissue is synthesized. Even most of the physical cells that make YOU today were not there six weeks ago.

Put simply, we possess a remarkable recuperative ability when properly nourished, maintained, and detoxified. While detoxification is a natural function, our elimination channels can become clogged due to toxic overload and poor diet. To improve their functioning we want to follow a comprehensive detoxification program. Such a practice, while unfamiliar to many, really is quite natural and beneficial. We regularly clean our homes, our cars, and our outer bodies. So why neglect the inner body? We have nothing to lose but our toxins!

Cleansing and detoxification are essential to healing the digestive tract and restoring good liver function. On some level, every cell is equipped with mechanisms to process and expel toxic substances, but entire systems are set up for powering more intricate and comprehensive detoxification. The majority of detoxification happens in either the gastrointestinal tract or the liver, which literally scrubs through our blood.

Two essential forms of detoxification we are continually aware of are the urine and feces we expel daily thanks to our kidneys and colon. But the body uses several other methods to eliminate waste that could be toxic to our organs. These include breathing (respiration), which facilitates the exchange of vital oxygen for toxic carbon dioxide. Even the small hairs in our noses (cilia) catch dust particles, and sneezing expels potential germs.

The lymphatic system transports toxins and excess fluid, and our sweat glands release toxins through the skin.

MYTH

Our body detoxifies itself and does not need extra help.

To achieve optimal cleaning results, we want to nourish and support all of our channels of elimination as often as we can. Doing this typically requires a few shifts in your lifestyle and diet, which help reduce your exposure to toxins and aid in your body's expulsion of current toxins camping out. Getting at those toxins is best accomplished through appropriate use of herbal cleanses, saunas, soaks, skin brushing, and colon hydrotherapy (the therapeutic infusion of water into the colon for the purpose of reducing its waste content). All of these forms of cleansing have been practiced historically throughout virtually every culture in one form or another.

There is no debate that we are equipped with magnificently designed bodies that can detect and process potentially hazardous materials and substances. The body has seven channels of elimination: the blood, the lymphatic system, and five organs—the colon, kidneys, lungs, skin, and liver. All have a unique role to play in getting rid of toxins, and all must be functioning optimally for effective total-body detoxification. But therein lies the challenge: the body burden we likely bear means these organs and systems require help to meet the demands we put on them. This is especially true if there is already a chronic disease state or if we are not taking in essential nutrients such as zinc, vitamin A, and selenium, which is necessary for one particular detoxification pathway. Most of us have hundreds of toxins stored in our bodies, all of which strain the natural states of our organs and tissues.

The Seven Channels of Elimination

1. **Lungs:** The lungs dispel toxins with every exhalation. Chief among these toxins is carbon dioxide, a by-product of respiration, the body's release of energy. The muscular contractions involved in breathing also help to transport lymph and blood, which also convey toxins. The lungs' lining of mucus and cilia (small hairs that capture airborne particles) help prevent toxins from entering the body.

2. **Liver:** In today's polluted world, health researchers believe the added toxic burden on our livers contributes to chronic fatigue, high cholesterol, irritable bowel syndrome, cognitive difficulties, and high blood pressure. A major organ of elimination, the liver serves as the manager of the entire detoxification process in the body.

3. **Colon:** The colon is the final place in the body where waste (food residue) travels before being eliminated. It is critical that bowel elimination happens daily.

4. **Kidneys:** The kidneys filter out water-soluble wastes from the blood that flows to them from the liver. These wastes are then stored in the bladder before elimination through the urine.

5. **Skin:** As a protective covering, it keeps toxins from entering the body. Simultaneously, because of its size and area, it actually eliminates more cellular waste than the colon and kidneys combined.

6. **Blood:** The blood that moves through the cardiovascular system is the key transportation system in the body, bringing nutrients and oxygen to the cells and flushing away waste products and toxins.

7. **Lymph:** Lymph, a clear fluid filled with immune cells called lymphocytes, moves around the body in a series of vessels that parallel the paths of the veins. Lymph delivers nutrients as well as collects cellular waste and helps destroy pathogens.

INHALE, EXHALE

The lungs go into action when we breathe, and their main function is gas exchange to the blood supply, which is connected to the lungs through tiny capillaries in the air sacs or alveoli. The lungs also filter and clear foreign particles that are in the approximately 10,000 liters of inspired air each day. Inside the lungs we have goblet cells that produce a mucus blanket, preventing drying of the lung walls and trapping particulate matter. The lungs also have ciliated cells, which beat at 1,000 to 1,500 cycles per minute in an upward motion. Together these two systems work to help clear particulate matter that enters the lungs from our air. Damage to either of these two systems can result in too little mucus and inability of the cilia to move, resulting in an accumulation of foreign matter in the lungs, some eventually making its way into the bloodstream. Toxic chemicals from the vapors, fumes, and gases we breath can also be transported into the bloodstream through the capillaries.

This blood from the lungs, which should just be full of oxygen, but now also has some toxic chemicals and maybe some particulate matter, gets transported to the heart. The heart then pumps this blood out to the rest of the body, including the liver.

Example: The dry-cleaning chemical perchloroethylene ("perc" for short) is a liquid at room temperature, but some of it evaporates and enters the air that you breathe. Exposure to perc is unavoidable for those who work in the dry-cleaning industry. Once breathed in, perc enters your lungs, travels into the alveoli (the final branches of the respiratory "tree"), and diffuses into the bloodstream. The blood now containing this chemical is shuffled off to the heart, possibly contributing to cellular damage within the heart muscle itself. The tainted blood is then pumped to the rest of the body, including the brain and spinal column. Effects of this chemical to the central nervous system include dizziness, headache, sleepiness, confusion, nausea, difficulty in speaking and walking.

The chemical also makes its way to the liver, where the liver performs its magic of trying to break this chemical down to something the body can dispose of, sending it out to the kidneys to get it out of the body through the urine. During this exposure time perc has been shown possibly to contribute to liver and kidney damage, liver and kidney cancers, and even leukemia. If a woman happens to be pregnant and is exposed to this chemical at higher levels or prolonged low levels, it can pass into the fetus, causing developmental birth defects. Now that California has banned the use of perc (it must be eliminated from all dry-cleaning shops by 2023), hopefully we will see a trend in its widespread ban across the world.

GUT CHECK

The small intestine is the body's major digestive organ. It is highly adapted for nutrient absorption, either directly into the bloodstream or into the lymphatic system through small blood and lymphatic capillaries connected to the tract. Lots of water-soluble toxins, like water-soluble vitamins, can easily pass through the intestinal wall into the blood capillaries, where they then enter the bloodstream. Fat-soluble toxins, such as fat-soluble vitamins, are larger-chain molecules and enter the lymph system. From there they are carried eventually into the blood in the chest cavity. All environmental toxins such as solvents, pesticides, food additives, and air pollution can be either fat-soluble or water-soluble, depending on their specific chemical makeup. Once in the blood, either directly through the intestinal wall or via the lymph system, the toxins will make their way to the liver. See the illustration on page 86 to put this into perspective.

Example: When you eat a mercury-laden fish, such as tuna or swordfish, it gets broken down and digested by our body's enzymes and bacteria. The absorption of mercury through the intestinal tract and into the bloodstream is relatively efficient. This mercury, along with the digested nutrients of your food, is then transported to your liver. As this blood is passing through the liver, the liver does in fact try its hardest to dispose of this toxic element by sending it out through the colon or kidneys. But, unfortunately, mercury likes to bind to proteins, especially those that make up our organs and tissues. Because of this, distribution of absorbed mercury throughout the body readily occurs via the blood and mercury passes quickly into organs, including brain and nerve tissue.

Symptoms characteristic of chronic, long-term exposure include nervousness, irritability, mood and personality changes, abnormal reflexes, speech disorders, and trouble walking. Once mercury is entrenched in body tissues, it clears very slowly, with a half-life of about ninety days (meaning it takes ninety days for half of the mercury to clear away). So if you stop exposing yourself to mercury today, you will not see immediate results. And in the event of mercury poisoning, you won't realize the benefits from ending your exposure for about a year, or four half-lives. This is actually a good thing because you don't want to rush mercury out of your body's tissues. It must be flushed out slowly from your body so you don't have acutely toxic levels of mercury dumping into your bloodstream and reinforcing more damage, let alone making you feel lousy.

FACT

Mercury is among the toxins that must be flushed slowly from your body. If you detoxify this heavy metal too quickly, you can experience adverse side effects that can be extremely harmful to your health. The mercury comes out of hiding and enters the bloodstream, where it can create trouble for your liver and other organs. This is called the Herxheimer reaction.

THE SKIN YOU'RE IN

The skin is the largest organ of the body, both in size and weight. It consists of two parts, the epidermis, or outer layer, and the dermis, the deeper, thicker layer. Inside the dermis layer is the subcutaneous layer that consists of fat cells, connective tissue, and large blood vessels. The skin plays a role both in excretion, the elimination of substances from the body, and absorption, the passage of materials from the external environment into the body cells. Conventional wisdom we carry from grade school has us believing that the skin is a protective sheath—a waterproof barrier to our vulnerable inner parts. But it is by no means an impermeable wall. To the contrary, substances can readily pass through the skin and affect our insides.

A small amount of water-soluble substances may be absorbed, but it is mostly the fat-soluble substances that penetrate the outer layer of the skin (this is most evident when you rub body lotion or oil onto your skin; lotions and oils are fat-soluble, which is why they get absorbed so easily). Fat-soluble toxins then pass into the dermis and into the blood vessels located there. Once in the blood, they travel through the blood vessels and eventually end up in the—you guessed it—liver.

Example: Transdermal drug administration relies on the skin's effective transport system. Drugs applied directly to the skin, usually via a cream or patch, get absorbed through the outer layer into the dermis and then into the blood vessels. From there the drug makes its way to the liver, where it can be processed and perform its function. Common transdermal drugs used today include nicotine and birth control patches.

Cosmetics and skin care creams that contain chemicals get into the bloodstream the same way. They don't just stay on top of the skin. Propylene glycol, for instance, is used in many cosmetic creams and makeup as a moisturizer or as an effective carrier of active ingredients through the skin layers and into the bloodstream. Although it is listed by the FDA as "generally recognized as safe," it is also listed on several government and environmental safety sites as being a suspected skin irritant that can also be toxic to the nervous, immune, and respiratory systems.

THE LIFE FORCE OF THE LIVER

Toxins that enter the body from the intestinal tract are transported to the liver, the largest and most active organ. We cannot live without a liver; it is a brilliant organ. So amazing, in fact, that it's the only organ that can self-regenerate, which is why you can donate a part of your liver to another person and it will grow into a full-size, fully functioning liver in each person. Fortunately, your liver is also the most resilient organ in the body, capable of continuing to work after injury and inflammation.

Although there are five primary organs of elimination in the body, both herbalists and practitioners of modern medicine agree that the liver is the primary organ of detoxification. It's the main hub where toxins are transformed, dismantled, neutralized, or reassembled to hopefully be eliminated through one of the four channels of absolute elimination: the lungs, the intestines, the skin, and the urine. If you have any weakness or debility in your liver, it will impact every other organ or system. The liver is so central to your body's overall functioning capacity that a basic tenet of naturopathic medicine is that many diseases can be treated through addressing the liver. In other words, if you can optimize your liver's function, you may help alleviate or cure other health problems either directly or indirectly.

The Life Force of the Liver: While the liver actually resides in the upper part of your abdomen on the right side, it's positioned here in the center to represent how fundamental it is in a variety of body functions. The liver, which is the largest internal organ, performs many tasks—metabolizes carbohydrates, fats, and proteins; stores substances such as glycogen and fat-soluble vitamins; filters blood; and destroys toxic chemicals. As a result, it affects virtually every other organ and system in the body.

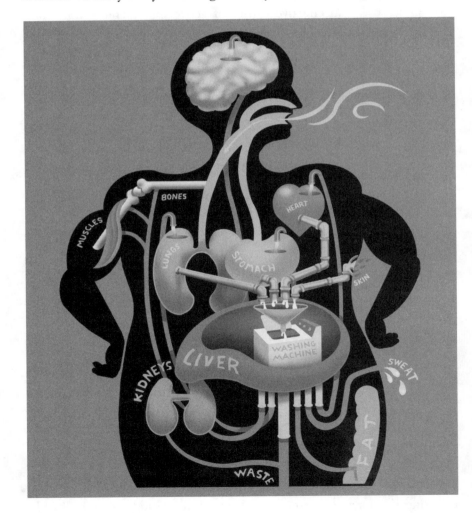

Love Your Liver

The liver is more than a washing machine for blood; it carries on many important metabolic activities—performing some five hundred other bodily functions, in fact (the most of any organ). It plays a key role in carbohydrate metabolism by responding to pancreatic hormones such as insulin and glucagon, thus helping maintain healthy levels of blood sugar; it effects the metabolism of fats, creating cholesterol and converting portions of carbohydrates and protein into fat molecules, which then get transported to fat cells for storage; it manufactures bile; and it plays a pivotal role in managing proteins. The liver can break proteins down into their amino acid parts, create vital blood proteins that aid in the clotting process, remove damaged red blood cells and foreign substances (like the remains of microorganisms), and convert certain amino acids to other amino acids that the body needs for operation. Furthermore, the liver acts as a huge storage unit, housing an abundance of substances including glycogen (for stored energy), iron, blood, and vitamins A, D, and B_{12}. In addition to removing toxic substances from the blood, it can also store them.

FACT

"Liver" comes from an Old English word meaning "life." Length and quality of life depend on proper liver function. A typical four-pound liver manufactures 13,000 different chemicals, maintains 2,000 enzyme systems, filters 100 gallons of blood daily, and produces 1 quart of bile daily. It sits on the right side of your abdomen under your ribs. You cannot survive more than 24 hours without a functioning liver.

Keeping your metabolic engines running and your body toxin free is a 24/7 job for your liver. Much like your heart's continuous beating, your liver continuously removes drugs, toxins, and hormones from the blood—deactivating and eliminating them. Remember, your body is in a constant state of renewal. New cells replace old cells. The same cells that comprise your stomach lining, skin, liver, blood, and even your DNA today will not be the same ones that make up these critical components next month. The same way your body prefers fresh cells, it also likes to keep churning new molecules and creating fresh supplies of myriad compounds, including hormones and proteins. This is why even "good" substances need to be broken down, reassembled, and either recycled or sent to the trash bin (i.e., properly eliminated). And it is your liver that holds the conductor's baton in orchestrating many of these perpetual operations.

A properly functioning liver is able to clear 99 percent of toxins from the blood before that blood is generated to the rest of the body. It does this through a two-step process called phase I and phase II liver detoxification. Every cell in your body actually has a similar biphasic detoxification process, but it is in the liver that this system is most active and highly intricate. The liver's pathways require specific nutrients to function properly, and if there is any mishap or missing nutrient in the assembly line as toxic substances get converted to less toxic substances for removal, your liver and subsequently your entire body may suffer. When the needed nutrients are adequately supplied, however, fat-soluble toxins (again, those that dissolve only in fat, and are commonly stored in fatty tissues and cell membranes) are converted into a more easily excreted water-soluble form. Once converted, they can then go on to the kidneys and bowels for proper excretion.

PHASE I AND II DETOX AT A GLANCE

Phase I in the liver is characterized by toxic elements getting biochemically transformed into a secondary substance, which then goes on to phase II, to be neutralized or made into yet another form that can be easily eliminated by the body. But these secondary substances—the intermediaries sandwiched between the two phases—can be more toxic than their primary counterparts. If phase II isn't working properly, your body may be worse off than if those original compounds had never gone through phase I. An accumulation of phase I products can be extremely toxic, such that the entire phase II system shuts down. This can happen, for example, in someone who has been exposed to toxins for a very long time.

Technically, the phase II liver detoxification process is called the conjugation pathway, but it's really a second wash cycle after the first one that entails a more rigorous process of breaking down the molecules further and binding them to specific types of proteins. These proteins help convert the intermediaries produced in phase I to water-soluble forms that can then be escorted out of the body through bile or urine (via colon or kidneys respectively).

Phase II actually involves six distinct pathways, one of which—the glutathione conjugation pathway—merits special attention. Glutathione is an amino acid, pivotal in the breakdown of carcinogens and the detoxification of industrial toxins; it also circulates in your bloodstream targeting free radicals, those loose cannonballs that destroy cellular structures and are thought to be involved in causing or complicating diseases such as cancer and heart disease. In your liver, this pathway's activity accounts for up to 60 percent of the toxins excreted in the bile. You can think of glutathione as one of the key, star players on your body's detox team.

The Importance of Bile

Bile is your liver's main vehicle for getting rid of excess substances, both good and bad; it's a complex fluid containing bile salts, electrolytes, old blood cells, cholesterol, excess hormones, and of course toxins. Once produced in the liver, it then flows into ducts leading to the gallbladder—much like tributaries leading to a river. This bile eventually makes its way to the small intestine, where it promotes the digestion of oils and fats. These can then be used by your body to build cells and bigger structures like hormones.

About one quart of this fat-emulsifying substance is produced every day and stored temporarily in the gallbladder, to be released when ingested dietary fat makes its way to the intestines. In addition to emulsifying fat, bile also lubricates the intestines, assists in absorption of fat-soluble vitamins, and promotes peristalsis (wavelike muscular movements in the intestines that keep your bowels moving on their way to the exit). Also, some toxins are carried out of the body in the bile through the stool.

Because bile links your liver, gallbladder, and digestive tract, people with liver problems frequently have gallbladder issues and vice versa. They are also likely to have digestion problems. You have probably heard about gallstones, which affect up to 20 million Americans and are twice as common among women. Gallstone formation is thought to be due to an imbalance of bile salts and minerals, dehydration, toxins, and excess cholesterol in the bile. In addition, a high-fat, low-fiber diet and pregnancy have been associated with gallstone production. When the delicate ratio that keeps bile in liquid form is imbalanced, crystals ("stones") form from some of those bile components. They can be a real medical problem, blocking the flow of bile from the liver and gallbladder, and sometimes obstructing the pancreas and intestines as well. These situations often constitute a surgical emergency.

Constipation Creates a Heavier Toxic Load

Constipation is the top gastrointestinal complaint in the United States. Few people realize, however, how this condition—especially when it's chronic—can amplify your toxic load. And so many people are constipated yet don't even know it! Being constipated is not just a backup of waste; it can lead to a reabsorption of toxins into the body and cause a further backup of toxins, which can then slow down the liver. Vegetables rank high on the detoxification program because they will help prevent constipation while also providing you with detox-supporting nutrients and the fiber you need to keep your bowels healthy and moving along your digestive tract.

A high intake of dietary fiber, which is the indigestible complex of plant foods found in fruits, vegetables, and whole grains, decreases absorption of toxins from stools and helps increase frequency and quantity of bowel movements. Indigenous cultures that have a high intake of dietary fiber invariably enjoy superior intestinal health and are virtually free of the diseases of modern civilization. As part of your RENEW program, you will focus on increasing your intake of fiber.

Signs of a Sluggish Liver

Your liver is responsible for producing most of the glutathione needed by the body, but supplies of this versatile amino acid can be depleted. Chronic illness, including liver disease and HIV, as well as excessive exercise, alcohol consumption, and exposure to high levels of toxins can all impair glutathione production and deplete storages. In addition to low glutathione, low levels of sulfur can also infringe on the liver's detoxification capacity. Sulfur is involved in another pathway that helps dismantle, process, and alter neurotransmitters, steroid hormones like testosterone and estrogen, drugs, industrial compounds, phenolics (benzene-derived compounds commonly used in plastics, disinfectants, and pharmaceuticals), and toxins from both intestinal bacteria and the environment.

When your body is deficient in dietary sulfur, your body cannot effectively detoxify certain substances. And some of these substances that rely on the so-called sulfation pathway to be broken down and eliminated can be highly toxic. Studies are now proving an association between dysfunction of this sulfation pathway and a host of illnesses including Alzheimer's, Parkinson's, autism, rheumatoid arthritis, food allergies, motor neuron disease, primary biliary cirrhosis, and multiple chemical sensitivity. In many people, the sulfation pathway in the liver is the weakest link in the system's chain of actions. Because the body cannot produce this molecule (sulfate) on its own, dietary sulfur is critical. Great sources of sulfur include not only eggs, high-quality fish and meat, but also an assortment of vegetables: onions, celery, kale, string beans, soybeans, turnips, radishes, and watercress.

A third pathway happens with the help of amino acids that the body can manufacture, and those include glycine, glutamine, arginine, taurine, and ornithine. Of these, glycine is the most important for neutralizing toxins. Even though your body can make glycine, it frequently runs out of available glycine. This is especially true if your body has a heavy load to detox, if you are not consuming enough protein-rich foods, or when you are experiencing an acutely stressful time period in your life that is taxing your body physically and essentially draining your energy reserves. In fact, any amino acid that your body can make (and requires to run efficiently) can become depleted through normal biological activities and added stress placed on it—both physical and psychological. In the Nourish step of **RENEW** you will consider supplementing your diet with amino acids that can help you maintain adequate levels. Many reports show that people who supplement their diets with a combination of essential and nonessential amino acids experience measurable improvements in their detoxification capabilities.

Blood tests can help indicate how well your liver is functioning, especially if there is a question about liver disease, but unfortunately these tests cannot show the true extent of your liver's functional capacity. For example, if your liver goes from operating from a full 10 (100 percent functional capacity) to a 7, this slight loss of function might not show up in traditional screening tests from blood alone. Such a slowdown in your liver's functional capacity, as well as its concurrent slowdown in detoxification, is called having a "sluggish liver." (There are tests available from several labs to help you identify this condition, which you'll find in the Directory. You can also ask your primary physician for help in getting these tests.) In this state, your liver won't process toxins at a normal and necessary speed, thus causing a buildup in your blood and potentially your organs. For instance, women who suffer from problematic premenstrual syndrome may have an unhealthy buildup of estrogen in the blood that has not been effectively removed by the liver. That excess estrogen can then aggravate her hormonal cycle and trigger more painful symptoms of PMS than normal.

There are many potential causes of a sluggish liver, in addition to the usual suspects of toxins like heavy metals. Certain medications, including cimetidine (antiulcer; brand name Tagamet), benzodiazepene-containing drugs (antidepressants and Valium), antihistamines, and oral contraceptives can all hinder phase I detoxification. Other inhibitors include grapefruit, the spice turmeric, capsicum of hot peppers, cloves, toxins from intestinal bacteria—even age can slow down your liver's first detoxification process. Doctors are now diagnosing more and more fatty livers (especially in children), a result of too much sugar and processed foods in the diet. A diet heavy in sugar and hydrogenated fats, the cornerstones of the processed foods that have infiltrated our lives, can encumber phase I detoxification and add to this vicious cycle.

The very toxins the liver is supposed to process are also contributing to a toxic buildup that inhibits the entire detoxification process. The liver cells themselves, which are designed to be champions of the detox process for the benefit of the entire body, are in effect damaged. As fewer detoxification enzymes get produced, the more difficult it is for your liver to operate at that level 10 capacity. So we see how damage can occur not only from the toxins themselves but from the amount of toxic buildup as part of our normal detox process, which also spurs the generation of copious free radicals. The harder the liver works, the more free radical formation, the more damage to the liver, and the harder the liver has to work to keep us healthy.

Signs of a Sluggish and/or Dysfunctional Liver

- poor skin tone and sallow coloring
- yellow-coated tongue
- dark circles under the eyes
- yellow discoloration of the eyes
- liver spots (brown spots on skin)
- acne rosacea (red pimples around nose, cheeks, and chin)
- itchy skin
- bitter taste in the mouth
- headaches
- moodiness and irritability
- excessive sweating
- arthritis
- flushed facial appearance or excessive facial blood vessels
- red palms and soles, which may also be itchy and inflamed
- trouble digesting fats (i.e., chronic indigestion, especially after rich meals)

The good news is that even a sluggish liver is still an effective one. Because there are six detoxification pathways in the liver alone, a weakness here or there is likely to be covered. An injury or illness can wipe out 90 percent of the liver's ability to function, and yet life will go on and the liver will recover. How amazing is that? For this reason, the liver is said to have a functional reserve. And it is this functional reserve that must be protected and that can be impaired by poor digestion, poor nutrition, a weakness in bile excretion, a genetic abnormality, or excessive exposure to toxins. It's critical that we care for and protect this indispensable organ as best we can. Yes, it's the most resilient organ in the body . . . but it is built this way *because of* how critical it is to maintain our life.

In the RENEW program, you will take an active role in supporting and optimizing a healthy liver detoxification system. This entails paying attention to diet and eating foods that will reduce your susceptibility to toxins' deleterious effects, as well as suffuse your body with nutrients or other elements that can enhance your body's normal detox processes. The liver depends on certain nutrients: the most important are antioxidants such as vitamins A, C, and E; the B vitamins; the minerals selenium and magnesium; and the amino acids glutathione, cysteine, glycine, taurine, and glutamine. People who are deficient in their dietary intake of fresh fruits, dark colorful vegetables, and cruciferous vegetables such as broccoli, cabbage, and Brussels sprouts could be lacking nutrients needed for proper detoxification. Those who are protein deficient may have a real problem with phase II detoxification, as this is where the amino acids are derived.

For example, while you may not necessarily know when you are running low on essential fatty acids critical to phase II detox, you can be sure adequate supplies are readily available by proper intake of foods or supplements high in omega-3 and omega-6 oils. Salmon, flaxseed, wheat germ, and the edible oils from sunflower, walnuts, and sesame all can give your body's innate detoxification systems a boost. To make sure you don't run low on glutathione, which is key to phase II, eating ample fresh fruits and vegetables will help replenish that vital supply. Phase II can further get a boost from broccoli, Brussels sprouts, cauliflower, citrus fruits, cabbage, and the oils from lemon peels. (Note that some of these act as phase I inhibitors but phase II enhancers.) As previously noted, eggs, onions, garlic, high-fiber legumes and grains all encourage optimal detoxification. Numerous herbs, spices, and vitamins can also improve the enzymatic activity of your body's detoxification systems, many of which will be part of your cleansing regimens. I will be giving you a comprehensive list of foods and supplements that will assist and maximize your detox.

FACT

Chronic alcohol abuse depletes your body of toxin-fighting glutathione, lowering your defenses against even the slightest dose of acetaminophen. Longtime alcohol users, even moderate social drinkers (three or fewer glasses of alcohol a day), who ingest acetaminophen are at risk for acute liver failure. The combination of alcohol and acetaminophen taxes the liver. When acetaminophen breaks down in phase I, an extremely toxic intermediary substance emerges that should, under normal circumstances, get processed immediately in phase II. But the alcohol intake speeds up phase I and creates a backlog of this toxic intermediary. Some health care providers speculate that alcohol-acetaminophen syndrome is the leading cause of acute liver damage in the United States.

BOOSTING YOUR BODY

I can't express enough how beneficial it is to nurture and nourish your body's incredibly powerful detoxification methods. The moment you decide to address this intricate, delicate system and lend a helping hand is the moment you choose optimal health and a better, more vibrant life. Such simple, concrete steps as eating cleanly, exercising regularly, and evicting as many toxic substances from your life as possible, begin paying off immediately. You'll likely watch unwanted weight disappear. You'll sense a diminishment in any medical condition you may currently have. And you'll feel more alive and be more productive throughout the day.

Remember, RENEW is based on the human body's innate (and, frankly, remarkable) capacity to heal itself, but biologically we are not all created exactly equal. Results will vary from individual to individual. Have patience with your results. Some may notice a change for the better in their health and energy levels almost immediately (a few days), while in others it may take more time. Everyone's body burden will be different, just as everyone's body (i.e., weight, metabolism, age, genetics, health status, and so on) will be different. All of this affects the impact RENEW will have on you.

Chapter 4 Summary

·

- The RENEW program is based on your body's natural capacity to heal itself. We cannot detoxify effectively on our own now that industry has given us too many foreign materials that our bodies don't recognize.

- The body has seven channels of elimination, five of which are organs (lungs, liver, colon, kidneys, and skin) and two are fluids (blood and lymph).

- Cleansing and detoxification are essential to healing the digestive tract and restoring good liver function—the two main hubs of detoxification.

- We further want to nourish and support all of our channels of elimination as often as we can. Doing this typically requires a few modifications to your lifestyle and diet, which help reduce your exposure to toxins and aid in your body's expulsions of current toxins hiding out deep in the body. As will be highlighted in the Detox Diet, foods that help optimize natural detox physiology include: broccoli, cauliflower, garlic, onions, egg, and most vegetables; high-fiber legumes and grains; and high-quality probiotics.

- As our chief cleansing organ, the liver dismantles or transforms both inner and outer substances so that they can be safely eliminated from the body. This is achieved through a two-step process called phase I and phase II liver detox.

- Because the liver is responsible for cleaning the blood that nourishes the rest of the body, any weakness or overburden upon the liver affects every other organ and system of the body. If the liver is not functioning to full capacity—called a sluggish liver—it can impact your central nervous system, your digestive system, your endocrine system, your reproductive system, and your cardiovascular system.

·

CHAPTER 5

STEP TWO: ELIMINATE TOXINS IN YOUR BODY

❧

The essence of the Detox Strategy is a collection of simple concepts and actionable steps comprising a multisystem approach for total body health and transformation. The goal is to stimulate optimum healing and function in all of your body's cells, and the result is a profound, total-body experience.

❧

Now that you have evicted many of the toxic elements in your environment to Reduce your exposure, it's time to address the toxins that have been accumulating in you for years. The E is about eliminating your present body burden. Remember, removing the external toxins to which you regularly expose yourself is just the first step in the RENEW process. The other half of the detox equation entails removing internal toxins that are already stored in your body. This chapter will show you the ways in which to enhance your body's natural detoxification process as well as assist in the expulsion of toxins at the cellular level and, ultimately, out of your body.

HERBAL CLEANSING REGIMENS

Herbal cleansing has long been used to naturally and safely assist in the body's detoxification systems. A tradition of herbal cleansing is recorded in the cultures of the ancient Sumerians, Egyptians, Romans, Greeks, Chinese, Europeans, and American and Asian Indians. The Chinese have a long and rich herbal tradition, dating back some five thousand years. They count their medicinal herbs in the thousands, as compared to the hundreds used therapeutically in Western societies. The therapeutic use of herbal preparations is also an integral part of Ayurvedic medicine, an ancient Indian system of healing that has its roots in Vedic culture. The American Indians also relied heavily on the healing properties of herbs. In fact, many of the over-the-counter drugs and prescription drugs in use today in our society are derived from Native American herbs. All cultures have traditionally used eliminative herbs that have laxative, diuretic (increases urine flow), diaphoretic (sweat-inducing), and blood-purifying properties to remove toxins from the body.

FACT

While drugs add to the toxic burden of the body, specific herbs can actually assist the body's natural detoxification process.

The heart of your herbal detox regimen is supplementation with herbs that will help all seven of your body's elimination channels (liver, lungs, colon, kidneys, blood, skin, and lymph) by means of several different mechanisms. Stimulating these channels naturally enhances the physical process of detoxification so that your body is able to rid itself of toxins without obstruction. Some of the mechanisms by which the recommended herbs enhance the detoxification process include:

- stimulation of bile production in the liver

- stimulation of peristalsis (wavelike movements in the intestines to move waste along)

- stimulation of urine output (a diuretic effect)

- hydration of the colon

- stimulation of blood and lymphatic circulation

- nutritional support to strengthen organs and protect them from toxic damage

- promotion of mucus discharge from lungs (an expectorant effect)

- eradication of pathogens (such as fungi, viruses, and bacteria)

- prevention of fat deposits in the liver

Numerous herbs working together synergistically provide the above effects, one of the most important of which is stimulating bile production and flow. You'll recall that bile is the fluid secreted by the liver and discharged to the small intestine, where it plays a critical role in the proper digestion of food, especially fats and proteins. It contains many used body substances such as salts, acids, hormones, cholesterol, mucus, fat, dead red blood cells, toxins, and other cellular debris. The liver dumps these toxic materials into the bile, which carries them into the colon so they may be flushed from the body. If bile flow is stagnant due to liver congestion, then the colon will not eliminate efficiently, and toxins will be retained. As they build up, your body will produce extra fat and retain water in an attempt to dilute toxins. The liver then becomes a key organ of elimination for the dual purposes of detoxification and weight loss. Liver support is central to any cleansing program. As always, you should consult with your doctor before implementing my suggestions.

WARNING

Do not use herbal detoxification products during pregnancy or nursing. There is little information on the passage of herbs through the placenta or breast milk and their effects on the developing fetus. Pregnancy is not a time to detoxify the body, it is a time for nourishment.

FOUR HERBAL CLEANSING STEPS TO INTERNAL HEALTH

To simplify the herbal detox process and maximize its effects, a four-step herbal cleansing program is recommended. The first two steps are total-body cleanses and I recommend doing them *at least twice a year*; this two-step protocol may be followed several times per year for optimal results.

You will start with a very gentle, basic cleanse for two weeks and then move on to the advanced cleanse for thirty days. At that point you will then have the option of completing one or both targeted cleansing regiments for the liver and heavy metals. If you choose to do these targeted programs, you will do them *after* the first two total-body cleanses, and you will do them in sequence (first the liver for thirty days, then heavy metals for thirty days). They contain herbal combinations designed to detoxify the body tissues more deeply.

The following are the four steps to take in order, with their individual durations:

- **STEP ONE—Total-Body Basic Cleanse**

    Duration: two weeks (at least twice a year)

    Formula: two-part (morning and evening supplements, described below)

- **STEP TWO—Total-Body Advanced Cleanse**

    Duration: thirty days (at least twice a year)

    Formula: two-part (morning and evening supplements, described below)

- **STEP THREE—Targeted Liver Cleanse (optional)**

    Duration: thirty days (as needed, *after* total-body basic and total-body advanced cleanses)

    Formula: two-part (morning and evening supplements, described below)

- **STEP FOUR—Targeted Heavy Metal Cleanse (optional)**

    Duration: thirty days (minimum); up to three months (as needed, *after* abovementioned cleanses)

    Formula: two-part (morning and evening supplements, described below)

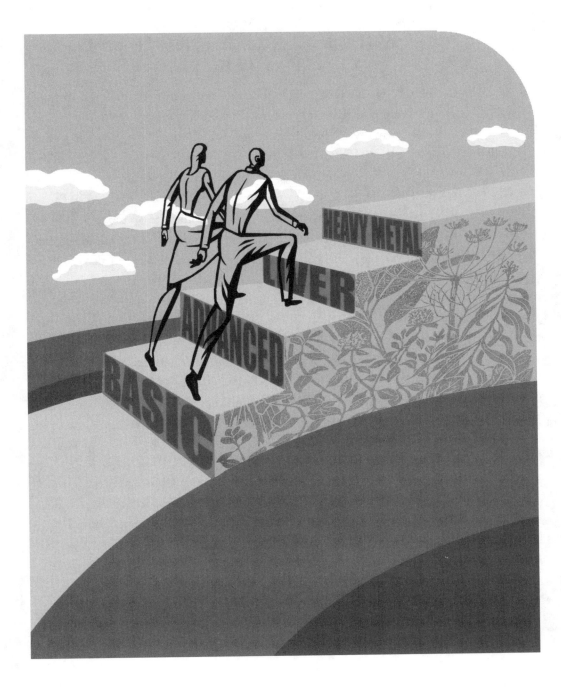

WHERE TO PURCHASE YOUR FORMULAS

Thankfully, we no longer have to create our own detoxification formulas from scratch now that high-quality supplements are available. You can find them in virtually all health food stores and some of the larger grocery chains such as Whole Foods, which carries a library of supplements (as well as other body care products) in its Whole Body section. You'll find a list of specific resources in the Resource Directory (page 265). But no matter where you live, chances are you won't have to go far to find herbal blends made specifically for the purpose of detoxification. Your local health food store employee who specializes in this section likely can also guide you in choosing the best one of the bunch. You may also find these formulas sold as kits—both the total basic and total advanced, for example, in one package with instructions. These two cleanses should take a month and a half to complete.

If you move on and complete both the liver and heavy metal cleanses, your daily active detox regimen will last at least three and a half months from start to finish. For first-timers and those who scored high on the test in Chapter 1, I recommend doing the entire program beginning with the total-body basic cleanse (it's best to start with this, regardless of how you scored on the self-test). Those who have cleansed before or who scored low may choose to do just the first two (total-body basic and total-body advanced) cleanses. However, if you feel that heavy metals, for example, could be an issue for you, then I recommend also going through the entire program starting with the total-body basic cleanse and ending with the heavy metal cleanses, especially if you have not done a targeted cleanse in the past. I'll give you tips on gauging your heavy metal toxicity below. I'll also give you leads for completing a specific mercury detox regimen.

Total-Body Basic Cleanse

Your ideal basic herbal detox program would consist of whole herbs. Such a product, formulated for people who have never cleansed before or who have not cleansed in a few years, would be a blend of safe, gentle and effective herbs that support all the channels of elimination and provide gentle bowel stimulation—including people who have colon elimination every day. This will prepare your body for more advanced cleanses. It would be formulated in such a way as to alleviate the "cleansing reaction" symptoms that first-time cleansers may experience while cleansing, and would be comprised mostly of organic herbs.

An ideal total-body basic cleanse would come in two parts, one for the morning and one for the evening. The morning formula would ideally consist of specific herbs to gently mobilize toxins stored in cells and tissues. The evening formula would contain some basic herbs to gently encourage bowel elimination. This basic cleanse would be a short one, approximately two weeks. Two morning-formula capsules would be taken before breakfast, then two evening-formula capsules before supper or at bedtime. Both are best taken with 8 ounces of water.

Following is a list of ingredients to look for. A formula that contains as many of these as possible promotes the safe elimination of toxins from the body.

Total-Body Basic Cleanse Ingredients

Morning Formula

artichoke	hawthorn berry	oregano
blessed thistle	horsetail	parsley
burdock root	kelp	red clover
dandelion	milk thistle	turmeric
echinacea	mullein	wormwood
fenugreek	nettle	yarrow
garlic	oatstraw	yellow dock
green tea		

Evening Formula

buckthorn	marshmallow*	slippery elm
flaxseed	rhubarb	triphala**

Total-Body Advanced Cleanse

The ideal advanced cleanse would be a blend of herbs and minerals formulated for deep total-body cleansing. It would work more deeply than the total-body basic cleanse, pulling out wastes and toxins that are deeply embedded in cells and tissues. In addition to cleansing the channels of elimination, the advanced cleanse would also provide additional nourishment and support. It would take longer than the total-body basic cleanse—lasting for thirty days with morning and evening formulas.

Following is a list of ingredients to look for; try to find a product that contains most of these.

Total-Body Advanced Cleanse Ingredients

Morning Formula

artichoke	celandine	larch
ashwagandha	chlorella	mullein
beet	cornsilk	milk thistle
burdock root	dandelion	red clover
bupleurum	hawthorn berry	turmeric

Evening Formula

cape aloe	magnesium hydroxide	slippery elm
fennel	marshmallow*	triphala**
ginger	rhubarb	

*Althaea officinalis
**An Ayurvedic formula

The morning formula of the advanced cleanse comprise specially selected herbs that target each elimination organ of the body to mobilize wastes, moving them from tissues and organs into the lymphatic system and bloodstream, to be eliminated from the body. Once the toxins are in the blood and lymph, they are eliminated primarily through the kidneys (in urine) and the liver (in bile). The herbs in the morning formula in the advanced cleanse function to

- **mobilize wastes and toxins stored in tissues**
- **stimulate bile flow in the liver for toxin excretion**
- **protect the cells of the liver from the effects of chemical toxins**
- **cleanse the urinary tract**
- **stimulate lymphatic flow**
- **boost immune function**
- **decrease respiratory mucus**
- **benefit skin conditions**
- **purify the blood**

The evening formula in the advanced cleanse will primarily target proper bowel elimination. These ingredients function to

- **tone and strengthen the bowel**
- **soothe bowel irritation**
- **lubricate the bowel**
- **decrease bowel mucus**
- **stimulate bowel movements for elimination of liver, digestive, and bowel toxins**

It is best to take two morning-formula capsules for the advanced cleanse with a glass (8 ounces) of water upon rising and two evening-capsules an hour before dinner or at bedtime with another glass of water for thirty days.

What to Expect During Active Detox

This program is designed to be gentle and should not cause you to miss work or live in the bathroom. Quite the contrary, you should begin to feel physically healthier and more energetic as the toxins get eliminated and the fog begins to lift. It is possible to experience a few minor side effects and general discomfort as those toxins get released into your bloodstream, including headache, cramps, and skin eruptions or irritations, but these reactions are generally short-lived, often lasting just a day or two, and usually no longer than a week. You will likely not notice any negative effects during the initial basic cleanse, which is relatively gentle as compared to the advanced cleanse. Depending upon your state of health, you may experience a range of results from the advanced formula, from weight loss and increased bowel movements to cold and flulike symptoms. If such cleansing symptoms occur, temporarily reduce dose to one capsule of the morning and evening formulas per day for a few days, and then resume full dosage in a few days. If you are concerned about any side effects or experience some and want advice or additional support, please talk to your doctor.

Adding the Other Elimination Actions to the Program

While you are doing these herbal detox programs, you will also want to be following some or all of the other recommendations, such as saunas, soaks, and colonics (as discussed later in this chapter) whenever possible. If you are doing all of this, plus herbal cleansing, you'll have a busy day. Since you'll have a lot to remember, you may want to create a detox schedule to help you stay on track with your regimen. You will have a lot of leeway as to when you do what, but as a general guideline, refer to the sample schedules in Chapter 8. This schedule also incorporates the other aspects of RENEW that will enhance the cleansing process and will help you tailor the recommendations from the entire RENEW program to your life.

Liver Cleanse (Optional)

We have already noted in Chapter 4 that the body's major detoxification organ, the liver, employs a two-part detoxification system that is dependent upon specific nutrients. When these nutrients are lacking or are in short supply and toxic exposure is high, toxins overwhelm the body, and the stage is set for illness to develop. For many people, liver damage from alcohol, prescription or recreational drugs, hepatitis, and repeated or acute toxic exposures, has created a need for extra liver support. Those with liver issues can benefit greatly from the use of an herbal liver-cleansing product. Ideally, such a product would contain a blend of specific herbs, antioxidants, and natural ingredients known to support, protect, stimulate, and detoxify the liver. It may be taken for a period of a month by anyone to help maximize liver support. As mentioned, it's best to do the liver cleanse after a complete round of both the total-body basic and total-body advanced regimens. This protocol will maximize liver function.

The ideal herbal liver-cleansing product would supply many of the necessary nutrients for phase I and phase II liver detoxification pathways, and contain nutraceuticals that

- **provide the necessary nutrients for both phases of liver detoxification**

- **protect the liver from chemical toxins**

- **provide antioxidants**

- **stimulate bile production**

- **provide important liver antioxidants and their precursors**

The recommended herbs in this ideal liver-cleansing product

- **stimulate bile flow to enhance elimination of toxins**

- **cleanse the kidneys for safe toxin elimination**

- **support the liver in dealing with chemical toxins**

- **scavenge free radicals**

Following is a list of ingredients to look for when seeking a high-quality liver detox product.

Liver Cleanse

Morning Formula*

alpha-lipoic acid	methionine	phosphatidylcholine
artichoke	taurine	selenium
dandelion	milk thistle	turmeric
green tea	N-acetylcysteine	

* This formula provides antioxidant and glutathione support.

Evening Formula*

Andrographis paniculata	*Boerhavia diffusa*	*Picrorhiza kurroa*
Belleric myrobalan	*Eclipta alba*	*Tinospora cordifolia*

* This formula increases bile flow.

Two morning-formula capsules in the recommended liver cleanse would be taken with water before breakfast. The evening formula would ideally contain important Indian herbs long used in Ayurvedic medicine. These herbs have liver-protecting and detoxification properties that have been documented in scientific studies. Two evening-formula capsules would ideally be taken with water before bed.

Heavy Metal Cleanse (Optional)

Since the Industrial Revolution, production and distribution of heavy metals have rapidly accelerated, so that the air, water, and topsoil of the planet have become permeated with them. These metals tend to persist and accumulate in the environment (and in our bodies!), for they cannot be degraded or destroyed. Today heavy metals are extensively used as components of countless consumer products, though the consumer is generally unaware of their presence in the seemingly harmless product. They are widely used in all forms of industry, agriculture, food processing, cosmetics, personal care products, household products, and so on. Most of us are familiar with what happens when we want a newer, faster computer or digital device that's been outdated by new technology. We have to discard the old hardware, which becomes electronic waste—and a main source of lead, mercury, cadmium, and chromium.

Today the speed of technology and the rapid turnover of electronic products in our disposable society makes for an ever-mounting pile of metallic waste to contend with. At the same time, our bodies are not evolving at the same rate to handle this massive accumulation from a biological standpoint. Once we breathe, swallow, or absorb these toxic elements (as with other toxins) they can accumulate in the central nervous system, the brain, the liver, kidneys, fat cells, and joints and greatly disrupt the body's normal functioning.

By definition, a heavy metal is any metallic element that has a relatively high density—at least five times that of water. Some of the twenty-three known heavy metals, such as selenium, copper, manganese and zinc, are nutritional minerals that are needed in small quantities to maintain health but can be toxic at higher doses. Other heavy metals, such as arsenic, cadmium, nickel, lead, and mercury, are toxic in even small amounts and represent a significant health threat when inhaled, absorbed, or ingested, for these elements cannot be degraded or destroyed.

Once toxic metals have accumulated in the body, they're not easily released from storage and flushed from the body. Although each metal produces its own set of unique symptoms at toxic levels, they all chiefly affect the nervous system, the production of blood cells, the kidneys, the reproductive system, and behavior. For this reason, heavy metal poisoning is associated with everything from depression and poor memory to insomnia, chronic fatigue, and kidney and liver damage. Moreover, heavy metals can disrupt normal metabolic processes and block detoxification pathways.

The more technologically advanced we get, the more metals we release out into our environment. I believe everyone would do well to complete the heavy metal detox regimen, even if you are not sure whether or not you carry a toxic load. For common sources of heavy metals, see the following list.

I believe everyone would do well to complete the heavy metal detox regimen, even if you are not sure whether or not you carry a toxic load.

Common Sources of Harmful Metals

- **Mercury:** Dental restorations (especially amalgam "silver" fillings), some vaccines (as the preservative thimerosal) and medicines, thermometers, old paint, pesticides, fish, flourescent lights, cosmetics, felt, fabric softener

- **Nickel:** Dental crowns and root canals, hydrogenated oils, inexpensive jewelry, batteries, cigarette smoke, stainless steel

- **Lead:** Old paint, automobile exhaust, insecticides, bullets, pewter ware, some hair colorings, tap water, batteries, pottery glazes, candle wicks, stained glass

- **Cadmium:** Cigarettes, batteries, automobile exhaust, pink dyes used in dentures, welding fumes, ceramic glazes, many art supplies, Teflon, fungicides, plastic

- **Copper:** Some cooking utensils and plumbing, gold dental fillings and crowns, insecticides

- **Aluminum:** Some drugs (including antacids), most baking powders, some cooking utensils, antiperspirants, cosmetics, foil, acid rain

- **Arsenic:** Pesticides, smog, tobacco smoke, a by-product of metal ore smelting and coal-fired power plants, wood preservatives in lumber and playgrounds, green pigment used in toys, curtains, carpets, colored chalk

- **Platinum:** Some dental gold, automobile exhaust

Below is a targeted program for detoxifying heavy metals, among the most difficult toxins to eliminate from the body. I've also provided information about a specific program you may choose to do called MercOut that involves more aggressive methods for drawing mercury in particular from deep within tissues where it likes to reside and out of the body with a trained doctor's supervision. People who go through mercury detox programs frequently report feeling more mentally sharp and energetic afterward. Many with neurological disorders in their families such as Parkinson's and Alzheimer's also gain peace of mind.

Progressive medical doctors have long used a process known as chelation to coax heavy metals out of the body. Chelation involves the introduction into the bloodstream of a substance that attracts and binds to the metals. Metals attach to this "chelating agent." Some nutrients serve as effective chelating agents when taken orally, which is what this metal cleanse accomplishes.

An increase in toxic metals in the body will displace needed nutritive minerals, possibly leading to deficiencies. Zinc and selenium in particular can become depleted through the chelation process. It is therefore necessary to include key nutritive minerals when undergoing a heavy metal cleanse. The ideal heavy metal cleansing product would be a two-part (morning and evening) formula containing key nutrients to restore normal metabolic processes that have been disturbed by heavy metal toxicity and important botanicals and nutrients that bind with and help excrete heavy metals from the body. For more about chelation, see the note on page 272. You may choose to go through a more rigorous form of chelation therapy under the supervision of a physician who can perform a "challenge test" at the start. This test involves introducing a specific chelating agent (i.e., EDTA, DMSA, and PMPS are the common ones today) to drive poisonous metals such as mercury, cadmium, arsenic, lead, and aluminum out of the body— from muscles, bones, fat, and organs. These powerful chelating agents will pull toxins into the urine, where they can be excreted and measured. Challenge tests help people determine their heavy metal load. But formal chelation therapy aside, you can benefit from a general heavy metal cleanse like the one below to bring your toxic metal load down gradually. These formulas entail natural chelating agents, including amino acids, vitamins, and minerals.

Following are ingredients to look for when choosing a heavy metal cleanse product.

Heavy Metal Cleanse Ingredients

Morning Formula*

biotin	manganese	vitamin B_2
boron	molybdenum	vitamin B_3
calcium	selenium	vitamin B_5
chromium	vanadium	vitamin B_6
copper	vitamin C	vitamin B_{12}
folic acid	vitamin B_1	zinc
magnesium		

* Do not start a heavy metal cleanse without first completing a total-body cleanse.

Evening Formula

alpha-lipoic acid	cilantro	leucine
bladderwrack	garlic	N-acetylcysteine
chlorella	kelp	sodium alginate

The morning formula in the heavy metal cleanse would be taken with breakfast. This would ideally supply balanced amounts of key minerals, replacing those minerals that might become displaced or imbalanced from heavy metal toxicity and through the chelation process itself. Two evening-formula capsules would be taken before dinner or at bedtime with water. Because the chelation process needs to be slow, I would suggest you do this type of detox program for a minimum of a month and up to three months if high toxicity is suspected.

A heavy metal cleansing product such as that described above would support the elimination of heavy metals without losing vital nutrients in the process. It would ideally be delivered in vegetable capsules and contain no binders or fillers.

The Mess in Mercury and the MercOut Solution

Your mother was right to be terrified of breaking the fever thermometer when you were a little kid and those little shiny, silvery beads would spill out. It may look harmless, but mercury is poisonous to every living thing on earth. Mercury contamination is so pernicious in America that health advisories for pregnant women or women who want to become pregnant are in effect in forty states. According to the American Heart Association, middle-aged men with high levels of mercury from contaminated fish have a 70 percent increased risk of dying from heart disease. Those mercury-laden fish absorbed toxins from industrial operations, as hundreds of tons of mercury are pumped into the air by industry, predominately through burning coal in energy plants. Mercury is also a disrupter of normal hormonal activity in the body, along with PCBs (polychlorinated biphenyls) and chlorinated pesticides that frequently get into this toxic mix. Swordfish and canned ("albacore") white tuna have taken a lot of blame lately for being the most mercury-rich fish, but other species of fish likely carry toxins as well.

The World Health Organization ranks dental amalgams ("silver" fillings) as the number one source of mercury in your body. The material dentists use to fill dental cavities is a mixture (amalgam) of metals, but it's at least 50 percent mercury. Amalgams are well documented to continuously release harmful mercury vapors into the brain, bloodstream, and other tissues. Galvanism with other metals in the mouth, such as gold or bridgework, can accelerate this process. Galvanism is a process by which a "battery" effect is created in the mouth when different kinds of metals come in contact with each other and saliva. This produces an electrical current that flows though the body and breaks down the amalgam, releasing higher levels of mercury vapor, and in some cases causing headaches, pain, and tremors. Dental bleaching can make this situation worse because bleaching agents can further increase the release of mercury from those fillings over time.

If you don't eat fish and have been one of the lucky few to have avoided cavities, you may still have mercury in your body as a result of any of the following other sources:

- vaccines
- fluorescent lightbulbs
- thermostats and barometers
- sports shoes that light up
- button cell batteries
- cosmetics
- disinfectants
- skin creams
- tattoos
- latex paint dated before 1991
- old chemistry sets
- blood pressure gauges

You can be exposed to mercury in a number of ways, and you may not realize it. Because mercury can be airborne, you can inhale it unknowingly (airborne mercury originating in Africa has been measured in the southern United States). Symptoms of mercury poisoning can happen at any time, as it continues to accumulate. Research shows that over time, mercury can quietly attack your heart, nervous and immune systems, including your brain and psyche, and disrupt reproduction and sexual performance.

One product I'd like to point out is Dr. Bruce Dooley's MercOut (www .mercout.com), which offers testing and products geared specifically toward addressing mercury levels in the body. The MercOut Detoxification Program in particular can safely remove mercury as well as lead and arsenic from your body. It's been designed by a medical doctor and the program is physician-monitored. I recommend checking out the site if you are concerned that you may have high levels of mercury in your system. MercOut also offers detection tests that can give you a more accurate result than what your regular doctor can find through blood tests alone. Because mercury is one of those toxins that hide in fatty tissues, it buries itself deeply within your organs and tissues—including your brain, heart muscles, nerve endings, and bones—and it can be difficult to gauge your mercury levels through generic blood and urine tests. MercOut has designed a program for bringing mercury out to measure it, and then employs special compounds with vitamins, minerals, and herbs for effective removal.

ADDITIONAL STRATEGIES TO ENCOURAGE TOXIN ELIMINATION

The following recommendations will enhance your natural detoxification systems—both during your active herbal cleansing program and as a routine habit when you are not on the herbal regimens. I encourage you to incorporate as many of these as possible into your overall program, and, once again, you'll find samples of cleansing schedules that include these ideas in Chapter 8.

Colon Hydrotherapy

Hydrotherapy, as its name implies, is water therapy. As a colon therapist, I have practiced colonics for more than fifteen years. They involve repeated infusions of filtered, warm water into all segments of the colon to remove excess waste that has collected and may not come out on its own. Colon hydrotherapy was first recorded in ancient Egyptian documents. It was also mentioned in the writings of the Sumerians, Chinese, Hindus, Greeks, and Romans. It is said that the practice of colon hydrotherapy in its most basic form, the enema, was passed down from the gods to the Egyptians. As with other practices that encourage detoxification, colonics have a long history.

Today colon hydrotherapists are trained to use massage techniques to help relax abdominal muscles and ensure that all areas of the colon are adequately irrigated and cleansed. Though the colon is filled and emptied a few times during one forty-five-minute session, there is no need for the client to leave the table to expel the water. The passage of the water in and out of the colon is controlled by the therapist who operates the colonic apparatus, while the client lies still on the table. As the water leaves the body, it passes through a clear viewing tube, allowing both client and therapist to see what is being eliminated from the colon. In addition to fecal matter, bubbles, mucus, and parasites are often seen.

There is no odor and in most instances no health risk involved in the colonic procedure when performed properly by a trained, certified colon

TIP

Some companies offer certain types of herbal products formulated especially for children. Do not use adult formulas on children or teens without first consulting with the company on proper dosage and with your child's pediatrician. Children under four should not use herbal detoxification products. Once again, consult their pediatrician about utilizing diet changes, probiotics, oils, enzymes, and fiber.

therapist. Therapeutic benefits of colon hydrotherapy include improved tone of colonic muscles, reduced stagnation of intestinal contents, reduced toxic waste absorption, and the thorough cleansing and balancing of the colon. It can also benefit your body's lymphatic system, for when the intestinal walls are impacted, the lymphatic system retains and continuously recirculates cellular waste. Your lymphatic system (your body's sewage system) becomes stagnant when the normally clear lymph fluid becomes thick with cellular debris, toxins, microorganisms, and dietary fats. Thickened, stagnant lymph contributes to fatigue, a vague feeling of illness, and weight gain—especially around the abdomen, hips, and buttocks.

Your colon can hold a great deal of waste material. That which is not eliminated promptly putrefies, adding to the toxic load of your body. Many people with "potbellies" may actually have several pounds of old, hardened fecal matter lodged within their colons. While colon hydrotherapy is not actually a weight loss procedure, it does often result in significant weight loss due to its ability to reduce the toxic burden of the large intestine efficiently. Furthermore, several ailments have been associated with colon toxicity. People with conditions ranging from allergies and acne to chronic fatigue and fibromyalgia may benefit from colon hydrotherapy.

Your cleansing, as well as your overall health, will be aided significantly by the addition of colon hydrotherapy sessions. Many patients have been able to overcome chronic constipation problems through colon hydrotherapy. Unlike chemical laxatives, which encourage dependency, colon hydrotherapy actually helps to tone the bowel, so that it resumes normal function. Hydrotherapy sessions can be used to "reeducate" the bowel to function normally.

The International Association for Colon Hydrotherapy (I-ACT), headquartered in San Antonio, Texas, is the worldwide certifying body for colon hydrotherapists. The organization works in conjunction with local municipalities to regulate the practice by establishing training standards and guidelines. To find an I-ACT-certified colon hydrotherapist who is using FDA-registered equipment, disposable rectal nozzles (speculums), and filtered water, contact I-ACT at 210-366-2888, or go to www.i-act.org.

Note: Although you should consult your doctor before implementing any of the regimens described in the book, you need to be particularly careful with respect to children. Do not schedule any colon hydrotherapy sessions for your children without first discussing with your pediatrician. Colon hydrotherapy on children should be done under the direct supervision of a medical doctor.

Getting at Least 35 Grams of Fiber a Day

A good fiber supplement is an important addition to any cleansing program. Fiber has been shown to aid elimination through the bowel and absorb toxins in the intestines, preventing their reabsorption. You will shoot for at least 35 grams of fiber per day through foods, but you can take a fiber supplement at bedtime that will help you reach that mark.

There are two basic types of fiber—soluble and insoluble—and both are valuable in detoxing. Soluble fiber (technically called pectin, gum, and mucilage) dissolves and breaks down in water. When it does, it forms a thick gel. It helps to think of soluble fiber as a sponge, actually soaking up toxins as it passes through your gastrointestinal (GI) tract and prolonging the time it takes your stomach to digest food so sugar is released and absorbed more slowly. It also binds with fatty acids, which are the building blocks of fats. In addition to helping regulate blood sugar, soluble fiber can lower total cholesterol and LDL cholesterol (bad cholesterol), thereby reducing the risk of heart disease.

Insoluble fiber, on the other hand (technically called cellulose, hemicellulose, and lignin), also known as roughage, does not dissolve in water or break down in your digestive system. Insoluble fiber passes through the gastrointestinal tract almost intact. Insoluble fiber moves bulk through the intestines and controls and balances the pH (degree of acidity or alkalinity) in the intestines. In doing so, it promotes regular bowel movements and prevents constipation, removes toxic waste from the colon, and helps prevent colon cancer by keeping an optimal pH in the intestines to prevent microbes

FACT

The fiber component of food is known as dietary fiber. Fiber is not technically a nutrient since we cannot digest it. While it contains no nutrients, the food in which fiber is found is loaded with them, and this is a powerful dietary connection. Where you find fiber, you find great health-giving nutrition.

from producing cancerous substances. In this way, it helps to think of insoluble fiber as a rake or broom—sweeping and literally pushing toxins through so they can be eliminated in the stool. Insoluble fiber also tones the bowel by creating resistance, giving the muscles of the colon some exercise by providing something for them to push against. This increases the minute muscle contractions necessary for good elimination, also called peristalsis.

Some Food Sources for Insoluble Fiber

cauliflower	potato skins	whole-grain breads
dried beans	root vegetable skins	whole-grain cereals
flaxseed	sour plums	whole-grain oatmeal
fruit skins	wheat bran	whole-grain pasta
popcorn		

Some Food Sources for Soluble Fiber

apples	cranberries	oranges
barley	lentils	peaches
beets	oat bran	peas
carrots		

Toxins that mimic the female hormone estrogen can have devastating effects on a woman's natural hormonal cycle, fertility, and general health. Many researchers believe fiber may help in fighting breast cancer. This theory is based upon the role of estrogen, and the evidence that shows how prolonged exposure to increased estrogen (and even progesterone) can increase cancer risk. In breast cancer, tumor growth is stimulated by estrogen. Fiber actually binds with estrogen and escorts it out of the body through normal bowel elimination. Hence, the theory goes that fiber can slow down the growth of breast tumors because it binds to estrogen and lowers the body's levels of this hormone, which can worsen tumor growth. This has been shown in numerous laboratory tests. What's more, fiber may help push out cancerous substances that have reached the intestines before they can cause serious damage.

It's important to get both types of fiber naturally found in fruits, vegetables, whole grains, and legumes. A blend of both soluble and insoluble dietary fiber makes for a brilliant orchestration of collecting toxins and carrying them out when you have a bowel movement. But getting your fiber solely from your food is very hard to accomplish. Rarely will you get enough fiber needed daily from these sources, especially in order to help detoxify the body. I would recommend a minimum of 35 to 45 grams of fiber daily during any of the detox programs discussed above. In order to get this amount it may be necessary to use a fiber supplement. Choose one that is organic and contains good sources of fiber such as flax, acacia, and gluten-free oat bran. Although some people choose psyllium as their fiber supplement, for many this type of fiber can be dehydrating to the colon, contributing to a more constipated state.

Saunas and Steambaths for Your Skin

The skin is the largest organ of your body, and a prime participant in elimination. Because of its size and area, it actually eliminates more cellular waste, through the pores, than the colon and kidneys combined. Sweating occurs naturally during strenuous activity such as exercise, exposure to the sun, or being in a warm room. Saunas (dry heat) or steambaths (wet heat) create sweat intentionally for therapeutic purposes. This "sweat (hyperthermic) therapy" not only releases toxins from the skin but also relaxes muscles, easing aches and pains. Releasing toxins via the skin through perspiration removes the load from the kidneys and liver, so those with impaired liver or kidney function may safely detoxify in this manner. It's imperative to remain in the sauna until sweating occurs. You won't get dehydrated, either, because you will respond to thirst signals afterward and drink water to replenish.

Raising your body's core temperature does more than just assist the detox process. It has also been shown to have a favorable impact upon the immune system. It is one of the few known ways to stimulate increased production of growth hormone, which helps the body shed fat, while maintaining lean muscle mass. Hyperthermic therapy also helps to restore autonomic nervous system function, which governs muscle tension, sweating, blood pressure, digestion, and balance. The autonomic nervous system is often dysfunctional in people with chronic fatigue and fibromyalgia. For this

TIP

To estimate the proper amount of fiber for a child, take their age and then add 5 to it. This will be the amount in grams of fiber suitable for that child. Example: a 5-year-old plus 5 grams = 10 grams of fiber daily. Most children could get this amount easily by including more fiber-rich foods. However, if your child does not want to eat fresh high-fiber type foods, then supplementation may be necessary. The best type of fiber supplement for a child would be a chewable combination including acacia fiber, larch, flax, or fruit and veggie fiber.

reason, people with these conditions can benefit from the sauna therapy.

There are two types of dry sauna: conventional and infrared. The conventional sauna uses electricity or burns wood as a source of generating heat. This type of sauna heats the air inside the unit to between 150 and 235 degrees Fahrenheit. You skin heats up by coming into contact with the hot air, and sweating soon follows. Because of the high temperature and the fact that conventional saunas heat the air, this type of sauna can be uncomfortable and difficult for some people to use effectively. If you can comfortably use, and have access to, a conventional sauna, we do recommend that you use it for our purposes; however, an infrared sauna is preferred.

Infrared saunas produce what is known as radiant heat. Infrared waves heat objects directly without heating the air in between. Because the air does not become hot, it can be used with greater comfort and for longer periods of time than conventional saunas. This allows for longer sessions during which you can sweat, shower off, and then return to the sauna again for intervals of sweating and washing off.

The heat of an infrared sauna also penetrates more deeply, although without the discomfort and draining effect often experienced in a conventionally heated sauna. An infrared sauna produces two to three times more sweat volume, and because of the lower temperatures used (110 to 130 degrees), it is considered safer for those at cardiovascular risk. These saunas have been successfully used by people suffering from sports injuries, arthritis, chronic fatigue, and fibromyalgia as well as other painful conditions. They accelerate the removal of toxic metals as well as organic toxins such as PCBs and pesticide residues—chemicals that are stored in the fatty tissues of the body and are not easily dislodged. The heat produced in infrared saunas is extremely beneficial for those suffering from such skin conditions as acne, eczema, psoriasis, and cellulite. The sweating caused by deep heat helps eliminate dead skin cells and improves skin tone and elasticity. Weight loss is facilitated through use of an infrared sauna, probably due to the increase in growth hormone that it produces. It has been calculated that one can burn 600 calories in 30 minutes in an infrared sauna. Health benefits

Some people falsely think excessive sweating is bad for you, but this couldn't be further from the truth. Sweating imparts numerous benefits; and if you don't sweat you will harbor more toxins.

can certainly be obtained in a conventional sauna or steambath as well, but the infrared sauna has a greater range of therapeutic efficiency, especially for detoxification.

The infrared sauna actually has an energizing effect on users, making them feel good as toxins are eliminated. Conventional saunas and steambaths are generally found in gymnasiums and health spas. Infrared saunas are more apt to be found in clinics run by holistic practitioners. People with health problems should consult a natural health care practitioner before using either type of sauna. (See the Resource Directory at the back of the book to learn where to find these.)

Rubbing essential oils on your body prior to using the sauna can help intensify the detox process of sauna. Try using oils derived from lemons, grapefruit, and juniper.

WARNING

Pregnant women and children under five should not use a sauna. For children five and older, consult your pediatrician before using a sauna. A child's core temperature will rise much faster than an adult's.

Soaks and Baths

If you don't have access to a sauna or steambath, you may want to do your own detoxification bath at home. This is prepared by filling a clean tub with hot filtered water (a shower filter or whole-house filter is recommended) as hot as you can comfortably tolerate. There are a number of therapeutic substances that can be used in the bathwater. One is Epsom salts, which contains magnesium to relax muscles and sulfur to aid in detoxification and help increase blood supply to the skin. A quarter of a cup of salts is a good start with a gradual increase to as much as two to four pounds per bath. My eucalyptus detox bath is a favorite. A recipe for this soak follows on page 122.

Another option is gingerroot. Ginger helps the body to sweat, so toxins are drawn to the skin's surface. To prepare the ginger bath, place half-inch slices of fresh ginger in boiling water over a stove; turn off the heat, and steep for thirty minutes. Remove the ginger, and add that water into a tub already filled with hot water. Other detox bath additives to consider include:

- **apple cider vinegar: increases blood supply to skin, changes its pH**
- **hydrogen peroxide: used in warm water (not hot), increases oxygen at the cellular level**

- clay: has drawing properties, alkalizing action
- oatstraw: good for skin conditions
- burdock root: helps the body excrete uric acid; useful when rashes are present

It helps to use a bath sheet or towel in the tub, soaking it and draping it over you as you would a bed sheet. Try to stay in the tub for twenty minutes, and repeat this procedure two to three times per week. For greater effects, add a cup of baking soda to the tub.

After any type of hyperthermic therapy (and during, if possible), be sure to drink plenty of water to replace fluid lost through perspiration.

Eucalyptus Detox Bath

1 cup	sea salt
2 cups	baking soda
1 cup	Epsom salts
2 tablespoons	glycerin per bath
15 drops	eucalyptus essential oil

Combine sea salt, baking soda, and Epsom salts in a bowl. Stir to blend. Pour $\frac{1}{4}$ cup or so into a running bath. Add 1 to 2 tablespoons of glycerin and 10 to 15 drops of eucalyptus oil. Store the remainder in a glass jar. Keep in a cool, dry place and use within two weeks.

Dry Skin Brushing

In addition to saunas and detox baths, toxins may be eliminated from the skin by brushing it with a special natural-bristle skin brush. This can be purchased in a health food store. (It's important to get the right kind of brush so ask at the store if you are unsure.) Brush the skin before showering or bathing, stroking toward the heart, gently but vigorously. This will help stimulate lymph flow, as well as remove dead skin cells. Remember, lymph flow is directly related to your immune and detoxification systems. At first dry skin brushing can feel uncomfortable, but it will improve as you keep doing it. The bonus is it will improve your skin tone, too.

Pure Air and Water

Remember to keep your air and water as clean as possible with the use of filters. Invest in a good-quality air purifier and change those filters regularly. Don't forget to change the filters in your air-conditioning unit as well. In the next chapter you'll learn some tips for jazzing up your water if you don't enjoy drinking plain water. If you use a distiller or drink reverse osmosis water, you would do well to go for a supplement that offers you added minerals.

Chapter 5 Summary

Step Two: Eliminate Toxins in Your Body

Eliminating toxins from your body involves specific herbal cleansing regimens and additional actions that support your body's normal detoxification processes. These include

- **Herbal cleansing regimens: The Four Steps to Internal Health**

   1. **total-body basic**
   2. **total-body advanced**
   3. **targeted liver (optional)**
   4. **targeted heavy metal (optional)**

      Formulas to cover all these cleansing regimes can be purchased at health food stores (or refer to the Resource Directory).

      During the active detox (while taking the herbal supplements), you should not experience major side effects that will disrupt your life. You can continue to go about your regular activities and work.

- **Additional practices to enhance detoxification**

   - **colon hydrotherapy**
   - **getting at least 35 grams of fiber a day**
   - **saunas and steambaths**
   - **soaks and baths**
   - **dry skin brushing**
   - **pure air and water**

CHAPTER 6

STEP THREE: NOURISH YOUR CELLS AND SYSTEMS

❧

One of the biggest myths—and arguably most health-damaging—we believe is that we get all the nourishment we need from the standard American diet. But the typical American diet is vastly unbalanced and contains insufficient amounts of nutrients required for optimal health. In addition, the soil and water in which a lot of our foods are grown are either littered with chemicals or so depleted of nutrients that they can leave the food depleted as well.

❧

Much of our foods are grown or irradiated in order to have a long shelf life. There is some controversy as to whether this process destroys the plants' natural enzymes that benefit our health but would also make the food decompose quicker. Most meats are laden with antibiotics, hormones, and chemicals that weaken our immune system. Most of our grains are processed to the point that they are devoid of the life-promoting benefits. The majority of doctors now agree that we can all benefit from daily nutritional supplementation, at the very least a multivitamin-mineral complex. For those of us who are hoping to achieve optimal health, a simple mass market multivitamin will not offer the needed nutrients for that goal.

In fact, surveys in North America show that the diets of more than 60 percent of people are deficient in one or more of the essential nutrients. Most surveys test for only eighteen of the forty-five known nutrients and use the standard Daily Values (DV), which are considered very low. Recognized as the minimal requirements for survival, they are inadequate to maintain optimal health. While these surveys look for common deficiencies such as iron; calcium; zinc; potassium; iodine; magnesium; selenium; manganese; vitamins A, C, E, B_1 (thiamine), B_2 (riboflavin), B_3 (niacin), and B_6; folate (folic acid); and iodine, they ignore equally important nutrients such as essential fatty acids and the amino acids critical to proper detoxification.

As you begin to remove toxins from your body, you'll want simultaneously to replenish your cells with as much good nutrition as you can get from both your regular diet and supplementation. This will help you fortify your immune system so it's capable of fighting the daily battle against toxins. Nourishing the body with healthy organic foods and supplements is something we should do on a daily basis.

In this chapter I outline a regimen of supplements and sources of high-quality nutrients to incorporate in the detox program. It includes my Detox Diet, which is simply a way of eating I hope you can adopt as a lifestyle for continued health. You will not have to follow a rigid and structured "diet" in the traditional sense of this word, though. Because the detoxification will happen primarily from the herbal cleansing formulas, it's important to stay focused on that part—plus the additional steps, including saunas, soaks, skin brushing, consuming more fiber and drinking pure water that will enhance the process. Changing one's way of eating can be a challenge, and especially difficult to do overnight. It usually requires a modification of habits long ingrained in one's lifestyle. This is especially true for people who regularly consume processed and fast foods, or who are not accustomed to purchasing whole, organic foods on a regular basis.

For this reason, I do not want to overwhelm those who will find it double-tasking to complete the detox supplement program *and* radically change their diet in one fell swoop. I don't expect you suddenly to become the model health nut. Remember to aim for slight shifts; this is not an all-or-nothing approach. If you are diligent about following the herbal formula plans and continue to eat as you would normally, you will still remove toxins from your body (although not maximally). Keep in mind that toxins will continue to enter your body, however, if your regular diet includes a significant amount of processed foods. In all likelihood, the detoxification from the herbal supplements alone will inspire you to make healthier food choices. You will find yourself automatically gravitating toward healthier options, and moving away from the unhealthy items that can sabotage your detox and your quest for vibrant health. As you begin to feel better and experience a shift in your body's energy level and sense of well-being, you'll want to continue to support that newfound health with a cleaner diet.

While I encourage you to do the best you can to adopt as many of my diet guidelines into your life as soon as possible, it's okay to take a gradual approach. Start on the weekend so by Monday you are already in the swing of it. I will give you a week's worth of menu ideas as a sample of what to eat during your detox. But there is no specific protocol that must be followed. The purpose of this Detox Diet is to show you how to nourish yourself well, whether during your active detox days on the herbal formulas or not. So, with this in mind, let's turn to my favorite supplements.

Remember, if you choose to remove sugar from your diet, it will take about two to three days before you feel better. By the same token, if you are a caffeine addict and choose to cut back (or eliminate) caffeine from your diet you may experience headaches for a few days. One option is to step down from regular coffee to green tea.

Virtually all of these recommended supplements can be found at your local health food store. They typically are located in the same place where you find your herbal cleansing formulas, so you can take care of all your detoxification product needs at once. For more leads on where you can buy high-quality supplements, see the Resource Directory.

ANTIOXIDANTS

Antioxidants are substances that will help protect your body from the damage of free radicals and may help to prevent such diseases as cardiovascular disease and many forms of cancer. Usually it is not necessary to take individual antioxidants; you can get a good antioxidant complex that includes the most noted vitamins, minerals, and nutrients known for their antioxidant properties. Look for antioxidants such as vitamin A, vitamin C, vitamin E, beta-carotene, lycopene, lutein, bioflavanoids, resveratrol, zinc, and selenium. You'll want a formulation that includes the full spectrum of B vitamins, including the activated forms of B_2 and B_6 (riboflavin-5´-phosphate and pyridoxal-5´-phosphate, respectively). You'll also want a multivitamin formula that includes vitamin D_3, and make sure the vitamin E is in the form of d-alpha-tocopherol. Avoid the "dl" form, which is synthetic. You'll want a high-potency vitamin C (about 1,000 mg) provided by ascorbic acid. An additional form of vitamin C, ascorbyl palmitate, which is a fat-soluble antioxidant, can enhance the formula.

You might also find antioxidant complexes with ingredients such as grapeseed extract, pine bark, blueberry extract, zeaxanthin, and astaxanthin. Astaxanthin, derived from algae, is believed to be several hundred times more effective than vitamin E in neutralizing free radicals.

Where minerals are concerned, in addition to the macrominerals (those needed in large amounts), such as calcium and magnesium, you'll also want to select a formula that has a wide range of trace minerals (those needed in small quantities), such as selenium, vanadium, chromium, boron, and iodine. Take these with meals as per label directions.

Why Vitamins and Minerals Are So Important

Vitamins and minerals act as catalysts to the digestion and metabolism of food. Vitamins are organic bio-molecules that act in small amounts as catalysts in chemical reactions. When acting as a catalyst, vitamins are bound to enzymes and are called cofactors. Because vitamins act with enzymes as cofactors, they make chemical reactions in the body happen—

including those that aid in your body's natural detoxification. Minerals, such as calcium, potassium, sodium, and sulfur, are also necessary to support biochemical pathways but, unlike vitamins, they do not contain carbon molecules and are considered inorganic.

Your liver as well as the rest of your body depends on a good amount of vitamins and minerals daily to support bodily functions. They are necessary for survival. When your diet is missing a particular vitamin, for example, over time you will suffer from a vitamin deficiency disease that may threaten your life. For example, in the past when we traveled by boat, limes were brought along for a vital supply of vitamin C, the absence of which can cause scurvy and eventually death. Knowledge of the necessity and power of vitamins has been widely established for decades, but more recently, researchers have discovered thousands of other phytonutrients that have an incredibly powerful effect on our health. It is as if we have discovered that there are really thousands of vitamins, not just the handful we all know about. These phytonutrients are found primarily in fruits and vegetables, as well as tea, nuts, whole grains, and legumes.

Some phytonutrients owe their health power to their antioxidant ability that destroys free radicals. Free radicals, as you have no doubt heard, are known to destroy cellular structures and are thought to be involved in causing or complicating diseases such as cancer and heart disease. Harmful free radicals can result from exposure to pollution and other toxins, as well as being produced by the body as it goes about its daily metabolic processes. You'll also recall that phytonutrients aid in the plant's own survival efforts. They use phytonutrients to protect themselves from disease and to boost their own immunity, and when we eat plants we gain some of the same benefits in those phytonutrients. That's one reason researchers believe organic fruits and vegetables are healthier—they are raised without pesticides, forcing them to produce more of their own protective chemicals. When we eat organic produce, we reap the benefits of the natural chemicals that plants have originally made for their own protection.

Let me give you an example. The phytonutrients in apples include chemicals called phenolic acids that defend the fruit against viruses, bacteria, and fungi. In this group of phenolics, a large family of chemicals that includes the flavonoids, is a natural antioxidant called quercetin that protects apples against disease. Research at Cornell University shows that consuming quercetin (which is mostly contained in apple skin and just below the peel) may lower the risk of Alzheimer's and Parkinson's disease by defending nerve cells against free radical damage. In addition, previous studies have shown that quercetin helps the body fight off cancer. Is this proof that an apple a day keeps the doctor away? I think we're just beginning to understand the power of these phytochemicals and there will be nothing but good news ahead. Where you find a healthy dose of phytonutrients, you often find a cornucopia of vitamins and minerals.

Calcium and Magnesium for Women

Women have an extra need for these minerals, so you would do well to add a calcium/magnesium supplement containing the proper ratio of these important macronutrients. Avoid carbonate forms of calcium (e.g., Tums), and instead look for a calcium-magnesium chelate containing a 2:1 ratio. This would be taken in addition to your multivitamin-mineral formula. Men need not add this combination supplement, but they can benefit from supplemental magnesium for better sleep, blood pressure, and bowel regularity.

AMINO ACIDS

These are the building blocks of protein. Our eyes look at food in different ways, but our bodies look at food in only one way. While we see a steak, a pizza, and a Caesar salad as different foods, our bodies see each as just a blend of energy in the form of protein, fat, and carbohydrates. Once we eat, our bodies go to work breaking down our meals into smaller units of energy that are transported into the bloodstream to provide the fuel we need to operate. From the time we begin chewing, digestive enzymes are secreted to break down our food into its component parts: Carbohydrates break down into glucose and other simple sugar molecules; fats break down into glycerol and fatty acid molecules; and proteins break down into amino acid molecules. Once this breakdown occurs, the resulting molecules are transported to the cells through the bloodstream and will either be absorbed by the cells for immediate use or stored for later use.

Proteins can be relatively large convoluted molecules, but their basic makeup remains the same—a collection of certain amino acids linked together to form a structure needed by the body to sustain life. The proteins used by the human body employ twenty amino acids. The body can make eleven of these amino acids; the remaining nine, known as essential amino acids, have to come from food. You cannot live for very long without getting ample protein, and especially without nourishing your cells with the essential amino acids they need to perform their specialized functions.

Dietary proteins are what help repair and rebuild muscle tissues, grow hair and nails, create enzymes and hormones, and maintain the health of your internal organs and blood. You also need protein to break down fat, where toxins may reside. What's more, some of the essential amino acids play a critical role in feeding the energy units of cells, called the mitochondria. If your body runs low on available glucose, amino acids can be converted to glucose and used as energy. Because protein is necessary to build and repair muscles, it's also critical that you have a sufficient intake of protein to improve recovery from physical activity and injury. Sometimes we can get amino acids in our multivitamins or in supplement form, but for the most part foods provide the wealth of amino acids we need.

Meat and other animal foods are said to contain complete protein, meaning they contain all of the essential amino acids. Individual vegetarian foods are technically incomplete because they are missing at least one essential amino acid. As a rule, though meats contain complete protein, they are not necessarily better for you than the protein found in vegetarian foods. Many types of meat are high in saturated fat, and all are completely devoid of fiber. Foods from plants are usually rich in fiber and contain vitamins and antioxidant nutrients that meat lacks. In the past, nutrition experts have recommended that vegetarians carefully combine different types of foods to ensure that they eat complete proteins. More recently, researchers have come to believe that as long as you eat a wide variety of fruits, vegetables, beans, nuts, and seeds, you are assured of taking in all the necessary amino acids.

Excellent Sources of Protein/Amino Acids

chicken	eggs	tofu (use sparingly)
turkey	pork (use sparingly)	fish—especially salmon
whey	beef (use sparingly)	(choose wild-caught)

Protein Foods to Avoid

processed luncheon meats	honey-baked ham fatty cuts of meat	liver

When you eat red meat, your health will benefit more by your choosing meat from grass-fed animals versus grain-fed. In recent times, since the introduction of factory farming, large cattle-raising operations have mainly fed grain to their livestock because it's cheaper and makes animals fatter and heavier. That means more profits for food companies. Consequently, most of the cuts of meat in supermarkets are from grain-fed animals.

However, the meat from grass-fed animals is more nutritious than the meat of grain-fed animals. It contains more conjugated linoleic acid (a component of fat that boosts fat-burning and the buildup of lean muscle mass), more omega-3 fats, and vitamin A. In addition, it has less fat, cholesterol, and calories. Farms that specialize in grass-fed cattle are also better for the environment. Cattle allowed to graze on large areas of land are easier on the land and pollute less than do factory farm animals.

Where chicken (and other poultry) is concerned, you'll not only want to look for the meat (and eggs) of grass-fed versus grain-fed animals, you'll also want to be certain that the animals are "free range," meaning that they roam freely in the outside environment, rather than being cooped up in factory farms where they are overcrowded and often subject to inhumane conditions.

Another option for a good protein source and companion for detoxification, especially for those who are vegetarian, is called "whole food multinutrients," a comprehensive vitamin and mineral supplement with an added food complex, amino acid complex, antioxidant complex, herbal complex, fruit and vegetable complexes. Look for one made from pea and rice protein.

Other important amino acids and antioxidants that you can find in supplement form to support detoxification include the following:

- **alpha-lipoic acid**
- **glutathione**
- **N-acetylcysteine**
- **glutamine**
- **calcium-d-glucarate**

ESSENTIAL FATTY ACIDS

Essential fatty acids (EFAs) are often referred to as good fats because of the healthy benefits they provide (they are a form of polyunsaturated fats). In fact, EFAs aren't just good, they are essential to supporting optimum health. And since the body cannot produce EFAs on its own, the only way to get them is through a proper diet or supplements, thus making outside sources of these fats essential. Essential fatty acids, especially omega-3, are needed for a healthy cardiovascular system, for proper nerve and brain function, proper hormone balance, proper elimination, and a solid immune system.

FACT

Fish oil is the best source for EPA and DHA omega-3s.

Unfortunately, most of our foods are devoid of these essential fatty acids, leaving the general population deficient as well. The best foods to get your essential fatty acids from are fish such as salmon, sardines, and anchovies as well as some plant oils such as flax oil.

There are three types of omega-3. The two you may be most familiar with are EPA (eicosapentaenoic acid) and DHA (docosahexaenoic acid), which are found primarily in oily coldwater fish such as tuna, salmon, and mackerel. Other than fresh-picked seaweed, which is not a staple of the American diet, plant foods rarely contain EPA or DHA. By contrast, the third omega-3, called alpha-linolenic acid (ALA), is found primarily in dark green leafy vegetables, flaxseed oil, and certain vegetable oils. Although ALA has different influences than DHA and EPA, your body has enzymes that can convert ALA to EPA. EPA, DHA, and ALA are important to human health.

Both omega-3s and -6s are vital to your health, but most people consume too much omega-6 and not enough omega-3. The reason for this is that most Americans have a diet rich in omega-6 source foods (fried foods, margarine, whole-grain bread, baked goods, and other saturated fats), and low in omega-3 source foods such as fish. Due to these eating habits, the typical American diet contains as much as 20 times more omega-6 than omega-3!

Eating a diet with significant amounts of foods rich in omega-3s can be highly beneficial. By increasing your intake of omega-3 fatty acids while reducing your intake of omega-6 fatty acids (especially from unhealthy sources), you will naturally bring the ratio of omega-3 and omega-6 fatty acids back to a healthier, 2:1 or (optimally) 1:1 balance. In addition to seeking healthy sources of essential fatty acids, I encourage supplementation with fish oil capsules. The purification techniques used ensure undetectable levels of mercury, PCBs, and other contaminants that can come with consuming tainted fish.

Look for a supplement that is either a balance of omega-3, -6, and -9 or for more therapeutic value, a concentrated, enteric-coated omega-3 supplement. If you are prone to burping oils, a good lipase-containing supplement (described in the upcoming pages under Enzymes) will aid in digestion.

The Benefits of Essential Fatty Acids

- nourishing active tissues, such as the brain, heart, eyes, and kidneys
- supporting healthy immune function and nervous system function
- supporting circulatory health and healthy metabolism
- supporting brain health and development
- promoting healthy hormone balance
- promoting a positive mood

PROBIOTICS

Probiotic supplements help keep a healthy balance of beneficial bacteria in your digestive tract, which is home to more than 500 different species of bacteria. Ideally, 80 percent are good or neutral bacteria and 20 percent are bad bacteria. As I already outlined in Chapter 3, there are literally trillions of individual bacteria residing in the digestive tract, with the majority of the population living in the large intestine. The two most prevalent probiotics are *lactobacillus*, which make up the majority of the probiotics living in your small intestine, and *bifidobacterium*, the most prevalent probiotics living in your large intestine. Good bacteria are critical in your body's ability to deflect incoming toxins and wrangle them to death or to proper elimination. So they are part of your Reduce and Nourish steps in the RENEW program.

FACT

Seventy percent of your immune system is located in your digestive tract. A healthy supply of good bacteria is critical to supporting immunity. An overgrowth of bad bacteria could suppress or overload the immune system. Keeping your bacteria in balance is essential to maintaining your overall health.

The Benefits of Probiotics

- promoting healthy immunity
- helping maintain healthy colon cells
- helping promote regularity
- helping manufacture vitamins, such as B and K
- helping manufacture some digestive enzymes that help the body digest food
- helping make use of nutrients, such as fiber, that would otherwise pass through the body undigested
- creating an unfriendly environment for potentially harmful bacteria and yeast

We receive much of the good bacteria we need through our diet. As we age, our body's stock of good bacteria decreases. Fermented dairy and vegetable foods such as yogurt, kefir, and sauerkraut are all high in good bacteria. If you want to increase the good bacteria in your digestive system, eat those foods and, most important, eat a high-fiber diet (35 grams or more per day). Why? Because good bacteria love to eat soluble fiber. When they eat soluble fiber, they multiply. When they multiply, they can crowd out the bad bacteria and maintain the proper balance. You can also support your bacterial balance by taking high-potency probiotic supplements that are formulated with the right balance of *lactobacillus* and *bifidobacterium*.

There are several critical, yet simple, factors to consider when choosing the right probiotic supplement. First, you should always look for high-potency formulas with significant amounts of both *bifidobacterium* and *lactobacillus* when selecting a daily maintenance probiotic; culture counts should be in the billions. These are the two primary probiotics in your digestive system. The second factor is your age. Remember, as we age, our probiotic population decreases. Choose a daily maintenance probiotic that is age-appropriate. The older you are, the more probiotics you need. Make sure that the probiotic you choose is either enteric-coated or delivered through BIO-tract tableting. Both of these methods ensure that the probiotics in the capsule or tablet bypass the harsh acidity of the stomach and are delivered to the small and large intestines, where they are needed most. If you have a particularly troublesome upper digestive tract, select a probiotic that includes glutamine, the amino acid that is the fuel for intestinal cells (make sure your upper-GI formula only is *not* enteric-coated or BIO-tract encapsulated; otherwise, it won't get broken down and used in the upper tract where you want it). And finally, if you are traveling, be sure to choose a probiotic that is shelf-stable and does not require refrigeration.

ENZYMES

As we have seen, enzymes are protein-based substances that play an essential role in every function in the human body. Those functions include eating, digesting, absorbing, seeing, hearing, smelling, breathing, kidney function, liver function, reproduction, elimination, and more. Like probiotics, digestive enzymes are powerful allies in your body's removal of toxins.

Historically, the best sources of enzymes have been from the consumption of fresh fruits and vegetables. Eating these foods on a daily basis is the foundation of good health. Even the food pyramid requires three to five servings of vegetables and two to three servings of fruit daily.

Unfortunately, too many people disregard these daily guidelines. The enzymatic level of fresh foods, such as fruits and vegetables, is reduced by long-term storage, pesticides, and toxins in the water and soil. As we age, the number of enzymes and their activity levels decrease. This is why supplementation with enzymes is helpful.

In the digestive system, enzymes break down foods by splitting apart the bonds that hold nutrients together—nutrients that the body will eventually use for energy. Normally, enzymes are present in raw foods to assist with digestion. However, many foods are depleted of their natural enzymes through cooking and processing. Without the essential enzymes needed for proper digestion, the body may not completely break down those foods to absorb their nutrients. As a result, undigested food in the digestive tract can ferment, causing gas, bloating, and other digestive difficulties. If you have trouble digesting certain foods, you may want to try supplementing your diet with some enzymes and see how it affects you. For example, if you tend to burp oils (say, after eating an oily fish like salmon), a supplement containing lipase with an enteric coating can greatly reduce this effect. Lipase is the enzyme needed for the proper digestion of fats. This enzyme is often added to fish oil capsules to help in the digestion of the oil.

A good enzyme supplement will not just substitute for the body in the digestive process. Supplementing with digestive enzymes will decrease the need for all of the pancreatic enzyme secretions to be active in the digestive tract. This will allow some of the pancreatic enzymes to be absorbed into the blood, where they can work on that portion of food that enters the blood and lymphatic system undigested, helping to break it down. Pancreatic enzymes also enhance the immune system. Look for a formula that will contain a variety of enzymes to address every type of food group ingested: fats, starches, dairy, plant, vegetable material (cellulose) and sugar. The ideal digestive enzyme supplement would be plant-based. Such enzymes are already activated as they enter the system and therefore start to work in the stomach, continuing to function throughout the body with a broad pH range.

FIBER SUPPLEMENTS

It can be difficult to get 35 grams of fiber in a day from foods alone (for a list of excellent sources of fiber, refer back to page 118 in Chapter 5). Ideally, you'll be getting your fiber from fresh fruits, vegetables, legumes, and whole grains. But to make sure you get your daily dose, it's helpful to have a good fiber supplement, shake, or bar on hand. There will be times when you'll want a quick, simple option for increasing your fiber intake; your busy lifestyle may prevent you from eating balanced meals every day, but there are ways to compensate when you have to grab a quick lunch or snack while on the go or even when you miss a meal. Depending on your situation and personal preference, you may want to select one or more of the following fiber supplements, bars, and shakes. These are delicious ways of getting your fiber in a super convenient and satisfying manner.

Chewable fiber wafer: Eating a couple of acacia-based chewable fiber wafers is a convenient option for supplementing your fiber intake when away from home. Ask your local health food store for help in finding these.

Clear fiber supplement: Consider adding another shaker to your kitchen table. Besides the salt and pepper shakers, you might want to keep a shaker full of an acacia fiber on hand. This clear, tasteless soluble fiber can be sprinkled on your food liberally to enhance the fiber content of your meals without altering the taste. Best of all, it contains no calories!

Bars: The high-fiber bars you'll want to use will ideally contain 10 grams of fiber (6 soluble and 4 insoluble) from milled flaxseed, oat fiber, and gum acacia, and 10 grams of protein from whey protein concentrate. Whey is an extremely high-quality protein, complete with all essential amino acids. Look for a bar that is sweetened with dates, raisins, and agave syrup and comes in a variety of flavors. Avoid any bars containing hydrogenated vegetable oils. Look instead for high-oleic sunflower oil, a stable oil that is rich in essential fatty acids.

Shakes: For a filling, meal-like shake, look for a mix that provides 10 grams of fiber (from acacia) per serving, and a decent amount of protein (around 20 grams) from a rich source, such as whey, as well as an array of important vitamins and minerals and an enzyme blend designed to ensure digestion of all classes of foods. Avoid any shakes that contain artificial sugar substitutes. Look for those containing tasty and nutritious natural sweeteners such as xylitol and stevia extract instead.

Note: If you are lactose intolerant, you likely will not have a problem with whey products, as whey is naturally low in lactose. But severity of lactose intolerance varies so much from person to person that you must be the judge. If your body responds to the whey found in most bars and shake mixes, opt for products that contain whey protein isolate. Choose whey protein products with less than 0.1 grams of lactose per tablespoon of powder. You may need to contact the manufacturer to find out more information on that, or speak with your health food store's representative, who can point you in the right direction.

During your active detox (while you are taking the herbal cleansing supplements), you will also take a fiber supplement at bedtime. Obviously, you wouldn't want to prepare a heavy shake or eat a bar just before bedtime, so this is when a fiber supplement you can dissolve in water is helpful. For a lighter shake, look for a "fruit and veggie" fiber mix that contains a fifty-fifty ratio of soluble and insoluble fiber. These mix well with water or juice and add a delicious hint of fresh fruit flavor to everything from yogurt and oatmeal to cereals and traditional smoothies.

LIQUID GREENS AND WHOLE-FOOD MULTINUTRIENTS

"Green formulas" offer combined extracts from various nutrient-rich sources such as dark green leafy vegetables, sprouts, sulfur-containing vegetables, and green tea. Liquid formulas are best. They can also include such ingredients as organic raw, uncooked aloe, which is readily absorbed by the body and is a nutritious whole-food method of delivering the nutrient-rich greens best.

Whole-food multinutrient supplements are also excellent ways of getting great nutrition on the spot without the fuss (usually sold as a powder to which you add water). These easily digested food supplements are loaded with protein, vitamins, minerals, herbs, and phytonutrients from nutritionally dense super foods that both enhance the cleansing experience and provide needed nutrients to support the renewal of a healthy body. Choose from a whole-food multinutrient from pea and rice protein if you are vegetarian.

Again, you'll find both liquid greens and whole-food multinutrient supplements at health food stores, or see the Resource Directory for specific suppliers.

THE DETOX DIET

The concept of nourishing your body is clearly tied directly to diet—what you eat. The foods you choose to put into your body are what ultimately nourish (or in some cases deplete) your cells. I just shared with you how high-quality proteins, for example, give you the amino acids you need to build and maintain bodily structures. Throughout this book I've been giving you clues to shifting a few dietary habits in pursuit of a healthier body that is less exposed to toxins and can better process those that do reach our inner sanctums or that have been with us for years. Some of these habits include moving toward organic foods that are fresh, clean, and whole, as well as avoiding processed, prepackaged, and refined foods. Choosing lean proteins that offer you all the amino acids you need to build and maintain numerous structures in the body—including those that are part of detoxification—is key. The result is an infusion of genuine nutrients that will aid in your digestion process rather than take away from or inhibit it.

Below are the guidelines for following my Detox Diet. Some of this information may sound familiar, as it will reinforce and reiterate concepts previously outlined. Remember, this is not a one-size-fits-all diet here, and there is no regimented diet plan for during or after you complete the herbal cleansings. I'll provide a sample menu for a week to give you plenty of direction, but ultimately you get to decide what you want to eat. All I ask is that you focus on staying on track with your herbal cleansing formulas and do your best to pay attention to what you eat and drink.

What follows are the components of—and the secrets to—a healthy eating lifestyle. Strive to incorporate as many of these suggestions as possible into your daily regimen. If you've been eating fast food every day for the last twenty years, I don't expect you to quit cold turkey. As with the other lifestyle changes critical to the entire RENEW detoxification program, go at your own pace and at the least, replace an old, unhealthy habit with a new one once or twice a week until you've made enough modifications in your lifestyle to put you on a path to vibrant health.

Use these ideas as recommendations that you can then tailor to your own personal needs, likes, and dislikes. You'll find recipes for a few of my favorite meals in Chapter 11.

Drink Half Your Body Weight in Ounces of Water Per Day

The human body is approximately two-thirds water by weight. The average adult has 40 to 50 quarts of water. It is necessary for most all functions in the body, including digestion, absorption, and circulation. Water helps detoxify the kidneys, helps dilute toxins, and is imperative for transporting nutrients in and waste out of our cells.

Seventy-five percent of Americans are chronically dehydrated. (This likely applies to half the world population.) In 37 percent of Americans, the thirst mechanism is so weak that it is often mistaken for hunger. Even mild dehydration will slow down one's metabolism as much as 3 percent. Lack of water is the number one trigger of daytime fatigue.

It is very important to drink enough water every day, especially to encourage detoxification. Carry your own distilled or filtered water (never tap water) and store it in glass, not plastic. Try to drink half your body weight in ounces per day. For example, a 140-pound person would drink 70 ounces of water. Adding lemon to your water is a great way to get the water you need and help alkalize the body, which is especially good during any detox program. Lemon is a natural stimulant to bile production and helps cleanse the kidneys. For people who do not enjoy drinking plain water, make a pitcher of herbal tea and keep it in the fridge. Try chamomile, ginger, or lemon balm. Celestial Seasonings

TIP

Lots of children do not like drinking plain water. Try adding a small amount of juice, such as fresh orange or mango. For teens, keep individual bottled waters in the fridge or on the counter, as some may not like water ice cold.

Red Zinger, or the berry teas are really good choices. You can make these in large containers to store in your refrigerator to have ready to consume as you would iced tea.

Another great option is to splash some cranberry extract into your water. Cranberry juice is famous for its antioxidant properties and support of a healthy urinary tract; its organic acids and fatty acids help keep bacteria from sticking to urinary tract cells. Cranberry can also decrease the incidence of constipation and urinary incontinence as well, especially in older people. If you don't have extract on hand, you can simply add an ounce of unsweetened cranberry juice (a good one is Just Cranberry) to an 8-ounce glass of water.

Detox Broth

During your cleansing regimens, you may choose to drink vegetable broth throughout the day, which will count as water intake. The recipe for this broth is in Chapter 11. It's the only recipe that is especially meant for use during your active detox.

Rally Around Raw Superfoods

There are many benefits to eating raw foods including the phytonutrient and live enzyme content. I am not suggesting eating raw meats but rather fruits, vegetables, nuts, seeds, and grains. There are certain raw foods that are either nutritious to the liver or will help detoxify the body in other ways. Making a point to include these foods into your diet can be very helpful. Here is a list of foods to include:

- **Raw beets:** stimulate the function of liver cells and encourage bile flow

- **Cilantro:** studies have shown it to be effective at chelating mercury and lead from the body

- **Parsley:** a natural diuretic, helps relieve congestion of the kidneys

- **Artichoke:** stimulates the flow of bile from the liver and gallbladder

- **Cruciferous veggies such as broccoli, cabbage, cauliflower, Brussels sprouts:** high sulfur content needed for liver detoxification, shown to speed excretion of cancerous substances from the body

- **Raw garlic:** its high sulfur content stimulates production of glutathione for liver detoxification; also has been shown to stop the duplication of cancer cells

- **Raw seaweeds:** contain alginates, which offer protection from environmental pollution; alginates bind with heavy metals such as lead, mercury, and other heavy metals; radioactive elements—strontium, barium, cesium—and are then excreted from the body

- **Raw wheatgrass juice:** contains high amounts of chlorophyll, which helps neutralize toxins and carcinogens in the body

- **Kale, chard, or any dark green leafy vegetable:** contain phytonutrients known to stop the damage of free radicals

- **Fresh-squeezed lemon juice:** alkalizing to the body, stimulating bile production and cleansing the kidneys

Why Raw Foods Trump Cooked Foods

Since meats are generally prepared at a temperature of at least 350 degrees and grains at 325 degrees or more, wholesale enzyme destruction occurs when these foods are cooked. Any processed foods, even uncooked, are devoid of enzymes due to the heat applied in the refining process. Freezing and refrigeration also have some effect on enzymes but result in only about a 30 percent loss.

When enzymes in food are destroyed or reduced, the digestive organs have to work harder to break down and process that food. Metabolic enzymes are then forced to perform this function instead of their intended job of healing. A deficiency of enzymes in the body is synonymous with a deficiency of life force. Nothing shows the value of raw foods more than the work done by the late Dr. Francis M. Pottenger. In 1946, he experimented with 900 cats. Half were fed raw milk and raw meat; the other half ate cooked meat and pasteurized (cooked) milk. During a ten-year period, he found that the cats on the raw diet thrived, while those on the cooked food diet showed all the degenerative diseases common in man. By the third generation, all the cats on the processed diet were sterile or congenitally malformed. Not only do we have more energy (life force) from raw foods in our diet, but our bodies are more thoroughly hydrated due to their high water content.

A diet of exclusively cooked foods forces the body to use its own fluids to moisten the ingested food, and therefore has a dehydrating effect. Dehydration is an important, though often overlooked, cause of many disorders, including constipation. Those with raw foods in their diet will require less extra water intake than those eating predominantly cooked foods. Any food prepared at temperatures less than 116 degrees may be considered "raw." Although conventional cooking requires much higher temperatures, tasty foods can be prepared at extremely low temperatures or without heat, using kitchen appliances such as juicers, dehydrators, food processors, and blenders. There are many fine cookbooks available at health food stores on how to prepare tasty raw foods.

Add raw foods gradually to your diet, especially if your current diet is composed largely of cooked food and/or you suffer from digestive disorders. Some people with inflammatory conditions can't process raw foods or, in some extreme cases, even cooked vegetables. Each person is different and must do what is best for his or her unique body chemistry. The simplest way to add raw foods is to alter cooking methods. As healing of the digestive tract occurs and as tolerance permits, fewer and fewer cooked foods are required. For example, the steaming time on vegetables may be gradually reduced so that they're eventually firm instead of soft, or they may be stir-fried to a similar consistency. Vegetables should never be boiled.

Experiment to see what you can tolerate. If getting enough vegetables is a problem, you may supplement with liquid greens or capsules. (See Resource Directory.)

Benefits of Juicing

The health benefits of fruits and vegetables have been recognized throughout history. In order to extract the nutrients the body must break down the fibrous plant cells that hold the powerful nutrient-dense juice. Juicing fruits and vegetables is a great way to unleash the benefits without all the digestive work. Not that the fiber of fruits and vegetables isn't wonderful for you, but you can also get a concentrated amount of the phytonutrients plants have to offer by juicing.

The benefit juicing has to offer to detoxification comes with the plants you choose to juice. Vegetables are preferable over fruits, as juicing many fruits concentrates the sugars found in fruit. Start with a dark green leafy base of kale or chard, and add vegetables such as beets, celery, and some lemon for taste or half an apple to sweeten it up a bit. It may not sound delicious, but it actually is, and it is cleansing and purifying to the blood and supports liver function. Chapter 11 contains my juicing recipes that are helpful during your detoxification program.

Most juicers are relatively inexpensive and are available in most big department stores such as Target and Wal-Mart. In order to juice wheatgrass you will need a special juicer. A wheatgrass juicer acts as a press that slowly extracts the wheatgrass juice from each blade of grass. Using a wheatgrass juicer is preferable because it does not destroy the enzymes with high speed. (Alternatively, you can find prepared wheatgrass juice at most health food stores, as well as chain juice bars such as Jamba Juice.)

Optional Brief Fast with Juice

I get a lot of questions about fasting, and how one can best reap the benefits of fasting for cleansing and detox purposes. You might not expect some of the reasoning behind being extremely careful about fasting, however.

Foods such as fatty meats, white flour, sugar, and dairy products can clog channels of elimination. There are also foods that build (make us stronger and more resilient), those that cleanse (relieve the toxic burden), and those that both cleanse and build. Proteins, such as meat and eggs, are the major builders. Most fruits are aggressive cleansers, while vegetables have both a cleansing and building effect on the body. Ideally, a detoxification diet will feature cleansing foods but contain enough of the building ones to prevent undue discomfort brought on by too rapid a release of toxins.

An extreme cleansing or detoxification program such as a water fast (where no food at all is eaten and no beverage consumed other than water), fruit diet, or prolonged juice "fast" is not recommended. While such practices do cleanse and accomplish the purpose of

TIP

Avoid all canned, bottled, and frozen juices. These lack fiber and can be loaded with added sug .. Stick with freshly prepared vegetables juices, especially the green juices.

giving the digestive organs a rest so that energy may be diverted to healing, they may also bring on a powerful cleansing reaction when toxins are released faster than they can be eliminated, causing a great deal of discomfort. A total fast can be debilitating for those with little or no nutritional reserves. A fruit diet, while accomplishing the task of cleansing, may also cause problems by eliciting a strong insulin response, thereby leading to blood sugar imbalances and other problems associated with carbohydrate overconsumption.

Most fruits, due to their high sugar content, also provide nourishment for any fungal organism we may be harboring, and can give rise to candida overgrowth and such attendant problems as fatigue, allergies, digestive problems, and brain fog.

For these reasons, I do not recommend anything more than a three-day juice fast during the detox program unless you are being supervised by a practitioner. If you scored higher than 25 on the self-test in Chapter 1, avoid fasting—especially if this is your first time completing a detox program. You can do a three-day fast the next time you choose to go through the program again in six months or a year.

To complete a three-day fast, follow the cleansing program as laid out in previous chapters but replace each meal with a freshly made juice drink (use the juice recipes on page 249). In Chapter 8 I'll be showing you how to put your RENEW program together, and there you'll also find sample schedules for completing the cleansing program with the fast included. A short fast of three days' duration, especially one that features freshly prepared vegetable juices, can be most beneficial to the body and is an excellent way to jump-start your cleansing program. Eat a light meal for dinner the night before you begin your juice fast. Try combining leafy greens such as spinach with a juicy green such as cucumber in a base of carrot juice. The addition of garlic or fresh ginger will enhance the therapeutic value (and taste) of your creation.

At the end of your three-day juice fast, introduce solid foods gradually, starting with the lighter ones like nonstarchy vegetables or citrus fruit. By dinner on the first day following your fast, you may add back starches, but wait another day before adding heavy protein foods such as meat.

Think Slippery Wet Rather than Dry

Avoid excessively cooked foods where much of the water is cooked out and the fiber is broken down by the heat. Eat raw, fiber-rich foods as much as possible, and eat foods that are wet versus dry; for example, chips and toast are dry, where as whole grains and vegetables are wet foods. Oatmeal is a better choice than dry cereal; and slippery flaxseed (when soaked in water), okra, and aloe vera are all examples of slippery wet foods that support a healthy gut and good bowel movements.

Eat Fruits and Nonstarchy Vegetables Freely

Choose fruits that have a low glycemic index, meaning they are broken down relatively slowly by your body so they don't rush into the bloodstream and cause a surge of insulin. Examples include berries of all sorts, pears, peaches, plums, dried apricots, cherries, bananas, apples, grapefruit, oranges, kiwis, and grapes. Minimize your intake of starchy vegetables, notably potatoes of all types, squash, tapioca pudding, and yams. Also limit legumes, which include beans, peas, and lentils. Beans in particular can be slightly challenging to digest, as they often cause gas. Beans are best consumed one type at a time, with as few other foods as possible, to avoid indigestion. Additionally, taking digestive enzymes high in amylase helps in their digestion. Soaking and washing beans before cooking eliminates enzyme inhibitors in the coat and makes for easier digestion. Similarly, sprouted beans are much easier to digest.

Any food that produces too much gas for you should be limited. Several vegetables, including mushrooms, broccoli, cabbage, cauliflower, Brussels sprouts, and other members of the *Brassica* family contain raffinose. When raffinose ferments in the digestive tract, it can cause gas and bloating. Sometimes digestive enzymes, taken before the meal, will help. Also, isolating these foods, eating them away from other foods, so the body can act on them specifically, or limiting or avoiding them altogether if they cause too much digestive upset, is recommended.

Whole Foods Versus Processed

Any food that is not "whole" is fragmented, and that fragmentation occurs as the result of food-processing procedures designed to extend shelf life and make the food look fresh and attractive. These processes include enriching, homogenizing, flavoring, preserving, milling, pasteurizing, coloring, irradiating, emulsifying, thickening, stabilizing, hydrogenating, and so on. While these processes may enhance the appearance of the foods and make them last longer, they do so at the expense of nutrients. Many food-processing procedures involve the application of heat, which destroys enzymes as well as many vitamins and minerals.

This is why focusing on fresh fruits and vegetables, preferably organic ones, is recommended when making the transition from processed to whole foods. Agricultural use of pesticides and herbicides has escalated wildly during a relatively brief span of time.

Wash organic produce in either hydrogen peroxide or a special "veggie wash" solution. This will help destroy any parasites. If fresh organic produce is unavailable, select frozen over canned. It has more nutritional value. Be sure to read labels, and avoid those foods that list chemical preservatives.

TIP

Avoid all processed foods made with refined cereal grains—commercial rolls, pasta, noodles, muffins, waffles, cookies, cake, doughnuts, pancakes, and crackers.

Also, as previously mentioned, avoid added sugar and artificial sweeteners, especially aspartame, sold as NutraSweet, which is a neurotoxic substance that has been associated with numerous health problems including dizziness, visual impairment, severe muscle aches, numbing of extremities, high blood pressure, retinal hemorrhaging, seizures, and depression. Sugars to eliminate include table sugar, honey, molasses, maple syrup, and other concentrated sweeteners. A moderate amount of the herb stevia may be used as a sweetener when needed. All sodas, diet and regular, should be strictly avoided.

Other foods to avoid are those containing partially hydrogenated vegetable oil. This man-made oil is found in commercial peanut butter, margarine, and most baked goods. Most supermarket oils are refined (unless kept in a special "health food" section) and not so labeled. Make sure the oil you use is labeled "unrefined" or "expeller pressed." Also remember to refrigerate them.

Refrigeration is actually optional for the tropical oils such as coconut oil, but a necessity with other types of oil since they spoil readily when exposed to heat and light. Air exposure will cause these oils to spoil, so they should be tightly sealed. You will also want to refrigerate nuts and seeds, and, since they contain enzyme inhibitors, which make them difficult to digest, they should be soaked overnight in water to make them more digestible.

> **TIP**
>
> Olive oil and/or coconut oil is suggested for use with cooking. Olive oil is also useful as (or in) a salad dressing. Unrefined extra virgin olive oil is the best choice. Flax oil is also good in a salad dressing, but don't cook with it because it is very heat-sensitive.

Most packaged grains found in grocery stores are refined. White rice is an example. Choose brown rice over white. Limit your intake of grains in general, which means no more than four servings a day (one half to one cup = one serving). Avoid wheat bread and wheat-based products; try sprouted grain or gluten-free breads. Food for Life has a great line of these products. Try some of the less familiar but highly nourishing whole grains such as millet, buckwheat, teff, quinoa, amaranth, spelt, bulgur wheat, and barley. These are all available, often in bulk form, through natural food stores. You'll want to "go organic" with these foods, as well as others, whenever possible. An organization that has worked diligently to increase awareness about the dangers of pesticides (as well as the hazards of food irradiation and biotechnology) is Food and Water, Inc., at 1-800-EAT-SAFE.

Go Wild

When choosing fresh fish, opt for wild-caught rather than farm-raised. Wild fish will have lower levels of contaminants, especially mercury, and be richer in healthy fats such as omega-3 fatty acids. The nonprofit Environmental Defense Organization has listed its "eco-worst" fish to eat: blue and striped marlin, swordfish, shark, Atlantic salmon, orange roughy, grouper, Chilean sea bass, and bluefin tuna. Choose smaller fish such as flounder, sole, pollock, and halibut instead. Consumer and public health groups indicate that virtually every can of tuna is contaminated to some degree, and fish-safety experts now think pregnant women should avoid canned tuna entirely because there's no way to know for sure which cans contain the least amount of mercury. Moreover, we don't know about the safety of even brief exposure to a fetus. (For more information on fish-eating safety, you may want to browse Environmental Defense's Web site and their "eco-best" and "eco-worst" fish at www.oceansalive.org.)

When choosing other meats, such as flank steak, top sirloin, London broil, chicken, and turkey—all of which are great, lean sources of meat—remember to go for organically raised, pastured animals (those that eat grass, not grains) whenever possible. Avoid the fattier cuts of meat such as bacon, beef ribs, chicken and turkey legs, fatty pork chops, fatty pork roasts, lamb chops, leg of lamb, pork ribs, pork sausage, and T-bone steak. Wild game can also be an excellent source of lean proteins without added fats and fillers typically found in farm-raised animals.

Watch Dairy

Avoid commercial dairy products, including milk, sour cream, buttermilk, cheeses, margarine, and other milk products. If you must include dairy in your diet, choose organic products that contain no hormones or antibiotics. Much depends on whether you are lactose intolerant, your blood type (i.e., people with blood types B and AB usually digest dairy better), and if the dairy is cultured, as in yogurt, or if the product is raw or pasteurized, since pasteurization makes dairy products more difficult to digest. This applies to milk and cheese. It is almost impossible to buy raw milk, unless you know someone who raises goats or cows. Raw cheese, however, is available in health food stores. Usually people can digest feta, cottage, and ricotta cheeses better than other cheeses. But again, much depends on other factors mentioned.

You can include butter and regular yogurt in small amounts—no more than one half cup per day.

TIP

Avoid or minimize use of table salt. Use unprocessed sea salt sparingly or try an herbal salt such as organic Herbamare (contains sea salt, kelp, garlic, onion, chives, parsley, celery, leek, cress, and thyme).

Slash the Salt

We need some salt in our diet, but we don't need to choose salty foods to get the proper amount. Try to minimize the following: deli meats, hot dogs, smoked, dried, and salted fish and meat, bacon, cheese, ham, most commercial salad dressings and condiments, pickled foods, pork rinds, processed meats, salted nuts, salted spices, sausages, and olives.

Select Superior Soy

Despite what current marketing campaigns would have you believe, soy can be a challenge to digest, and you'll recall from Chapter 3 that some soy products may come from a genetically modified (GM) food source. Uncultured soy products, which include texturized vegetable protein (TVP), isolated soy protein, soy protein isolates, soy milk, soy flour, soy nuts, and edamame bean, pose a digestive challenge for some people. Soy that has been fermented or broken down by beneficial bacteria (similar to how cabbage becomes sauerkraut, or milk becomes yogurt) is the least challenging to people's digestion. These forms include tempeh, miso, and natto, which are superior to other forms of soy. Tofu is not cultured, but is precipitated into a curd from soy milk and is a more concentrated protein than other forms of soybean preparations; it can be better digested if eaten with vegetables, or eaten in a soup broth.

Soy imparts excellent health benefits due to their isoflavones, which is why you should consider consuming non-GMO, cultured forms of soy (i.e., miso, tempeh, and natto) in moderation. Isoflavones are weak phytoestrogens that have the ability to bind to estrogen receptors and reduce total cholesterol—lowing LDL and possibly increasing HDL (the good cholesterol that helps keep LDL in check). Isoflavones may also help maintain bone mass, reduce hot flashes in postmenopausal women, and lower the risk of cardiovascular disease.

Drink Clean

Avoid or limit coffee and tea. Choose organic, decaffeinated coffee and/or herbal teas instead. Try drinking products that have been decaffeinated by a chemical-free water process, such as the Swiss Water Process; otherwise, decaf drinks can be yet another source of toxins. I recommend switching to green tea if you must have your daily cup. Avoid or significantly minimize alcoholic beverages.

Time Management and Meal Planning

Meal planning and time management are key components in creating a healthy eating plan, for food selection is of paramount importance in achieving vibrant health. The first step is reviewing your lifestyle and determining how healthy foods can be integrated into it. Plan your meals for one week before visiting the market. When possible, plan lunches for you and your children ahead of time. Typical school lunches are not very nourishing, and neither are the fast foods so popular at lunch. Ideally, meal planning for the coming week would be done on the weekend or on your day off. Selections would best be written down for better organizing and planning. Make grocery shopping a part of your weekly routine, and make a habit of washing fruits and vegetables thoroughly before storing them. This saves time during the week when time is of the essence. If a weekly plan includes eating at restaurants, then select only those that offer healthy options.

Local markets and health food stores offer the best choices of quality foods to be prepared at home. Look for stores that stock organic fruits, vegetables, and meats. You'll want to discard any unhealthy foods—sugar, refined starches, soda pop, et cetera—that may have been purchased before starting your healthy diet.

Looking at what you will need in terms of appliances will save you time in the kitchen. One of the most important time-saving appliances is a slow cooker (brand name Crock-Pot). With this method, foods are cooked slowly throughout the day and are ready to serve when you get home from work.

Balancing pH

What's important to know about pH is that most grains, all meats, and sugary foods are acid-forming in the body, while most fruits (even citrus) and vegetables are alkaline-forming (though they may be acid in their raw, undigested form). The consensus among experts in the natural health field seems to be that the ideal diet would consist of 80 percent alkaline-forming foods and 20 percent acid-forming foods. That means more fruits and vegetables should be eaten than meats and grains. The SAD (Standard American Diet) is backward, with emphasis on starchy carbohydrates and meat. This imbalance can be corrected by adding fruits and vegetables to the diet while limiting starchy carbohydrates.

A green salad at least once per day and at least one cooked green vegetable daily, gradually adding more greens, will achieve an ideal diet. In addition to increasing the number of salads and vegetables eaten, you may wish to add green drinks and/or capsules to your daily routine. (See Resource Directory for specific products.) For the sample menu that follows, remember that the recipes can be found starting on page 241.

SAMPLE MENUS FOR A WEEK

Day 1:   B   2 to 3 scrambled eggs with 2 to 4 vegetables of choice, cooked in extra virgin olive oil and topped with salsa and avocado; multigrain toast with organic butter or almond butter

L   Endive Salad*

D   Roasted Blackened Salmon*; Steamed Mediterranean Asparagus*; and acorn squash

Snacks: Citrus Cocktail or other juice drink*; fiber bar or shake

Day 2:   B   Nutty Rice Porridge*

L   Large garden salad with mixed greens and several vegetables (carrots, radishes, raw beets, sweet peppers); turkey or chicken slices; vinaigrette dressing; raw wheatgrass juice

D   Dover Sole Roll-ups*

Snacks: Celery sticks stuffed with natural peanut or almond butter; Pineapple Cooler or other juice drink*

Day 3:   B   Eggless Veggie Omelet*

L   Cup of soup of your choice and small spinach salad or baby greens salad with chickpeas and grilled chicken (choose a clear-based soup, not cream-based)

D   Pasta marinara or chicken cacciatore with sautéed vegetables

Snacks: Fresh Garden Tonic or other juice drink*; fiber bar or shake

Day 4:   B   Digestive Cocktail* and bowl of oatmeal topped with raspberries, raisins, and walnuts

L   Grilled Tempeh with Mixed Greens*; raw wheatgrass juice

D   Any baked or broiled fish with Almond Brown Rice with Orange*; sautéed kale, or steamed vegetable of your choice

Snacks: Tropical Spritzer or other juice drink*; fresh fruit or steamed artichoke

See recipe

Day 5: B Multigrain French toast with Greek-style yogurt and bananas

L Endive Salad*

D Organic, lean ground chicken or turkey pan-fried in dash of olive oil with medley of vegetables and pine nuts, rolled up in tortilla; top with salsa and avocado

Snacks: Sweet Body Cleanse or other juice drink*; fiber bar, shake, or fresh fruit

Day 6: B Brown Rice Breakfast Cereal* or 2 to 3 eggs scrambled with 2 to 3 vegetables of your choice, cooked in extra virgin olive oil and topped with cilantro and salsa

L Minestrone or vegetable soup with large garden salad; raw wheatgrass juice

D Stir-fry chicken with asparagus and garlic; brown rice

Snacks: Red Detox juice drink*; fiber bar or shake; carrot sticks dipped in hummus

Day 7: B Eggless Veggie Omelet* or buckwheat pancakes with blueberries and raspberries

L Large garden salad with mixed greens and several vegetables (carrots, radishes, sweet peppers); turkey or chicken slices; vinaigrette dressing

D Any baked or broiled fish with brown rice and steamed vegetable of your choice

Snacks: Basic Blend or other juice drink*; fiber bar or shake

See recipe

Beverage ideas:

Choose plain (filtered) water, or drink the detox broth throughout the day. You can spice up your water with the juice of a lemon, lime, or orange (or add wedges of these fruits). Try adding cucumber slices or a splash of pure (nothing added) cranberry or pomegranate juice to sparkling water. Other options: green tea and hot or cold herbal tea.

Final Tips

Here are some additional tips to bear in mind at your next meal:

- Watch your portions: Because overeating can put stress on the digestive organs, infringe on normal detoxification pathways, and lead to obesity and disease, many of us would do well to address the issue of portion control.

- Eat s-l-o-w-l-y: This will help you to chew your food properly before sending it on to the stomach for further digestion. It will also help you to control your portions better and keep you from overeating. It takes time for your brain to receive signals that you are full. When you eat slowly, you can enjoy your meal maximally and give your body the time it needs to digest efficiently.

- Avoid drinking large amounts of liquid with your meals or immediately afterward. This can interfere with digestion.

- Stressed out? Before sitting down to eat, spend five or ten minutes doing something to unwind and to take your mind off stressful thoughts. Taking a few minutes to sit in silence and breathe deeply can work wonders on lowering your stress level a notch or two.

Chapter 6 Summary

- More than 60 percent of Americans are deficient in one or more essential nutrients. The average diet further adds to our toxic load through refined sugars, additives, preservatives, and exposure to pesticides. Eating closer to nature—choosing organically grown foods and high-quality sources of proteins and other nutrients—will support our bodies' detoxification processes.

- Supplements can support your detox program and your path to vibrant health.
  - **Supplements Highly Recommended for Everyone**
    multivitamin and mineral formula (source of antioxidants)
    omega-3 fatty acids (fish oil)
    calcium and magnesium (for women)
    magnesium (for men)
    probiotics
    fiber (chewable fiber wafers, clear fiber in shaker, bars, and shakes)

  - **Optional Supplements as Needed**
    amino acids
    digestive enzymes
    liquid greens
    whole-food multinutrient

- The Detox Diet is a collection of tips on healthier, cleaner eating that you would do well to incorporate into your life as much as possible. It strongly encourages the following:
  - water (not tap)
  - raw foods
  - juicing
  - fruits and nonstarchy vegetables
  - whole rather than processed foods
  - wild fish and game

- The Detox Diet discourages commercial dairy, salt, caffeine, and alcohol.

CHAPTER 7

STEP FOUR: ENERGIZE YOUR BODY, MIND, AND SPIRIT

❧

When you think energize, think exercise. Think movement. Think circulation. Think vitality. And think detox. Getting physical and upping your cardiac output—from taking a brisk walk to activities like running, swimming, and cycling—is one of the greatest ways to naturally cleanse the blood and all body tissues. Put simply, exercise is body purification.

❧

In this brief chapter, I'm going to share some of my secret techniques to using exercise for purposes of complementing your detoxification program. Certainly, we all may have unique reasons or motivators for working out— to become more fit, to train for an athletic event, to lower our resting heart rate or address another medical concern, to lose weight, to unwind and destress, and so on. But when it comes to assisting the body's natural detoxification systems, a few exercises uniquely apply here. I should also point out that no matter which physical activities you ultimately choose to do, most all of them cause you to sweat, which is important to the entire detoxification process as one of the main channels of detox. I'll also give you hints on rest and relaxation, which should be part of your path to optimum wellness.

THE MAGIC OF DEEP BREATHING

Before we get to the sweat factor, I want to reiterate an often underestimated outcome to moving your body physically and its related benefits for detox: deep breathing. It can be an exercise for relaxation and meditation in itself, but as you commence a more active lifestyle, I want you to be thinking about your breathing in particular. Here's why.

The mere act of breathing in and out stimulates the flow of lymph through the body. You'll recall that lymph is the clear fluid filled with immune cells that moves around the body in a series of vessels, delivering nutrients and collecting cellular waste while helping to destroy pathogens. The deeper you breathe, the more you can achieve this effect. It has long been known that exercise stimulates this movement of lymphatic fluid, but the role of breathing wasn't entirely recognized until technology provided the means to photograph lymph flow. This direct observation shows that deep breathing causes the lymph to shoot through the capillaries like a geyser.

Breathing deeply helps eliminate poisons (yes, toxins included) from the cells, and also enhances immunity, since the lymphatic system is actually part of the immune system. While the heart is the pump for the vascular system, the lymphatic system has no real pump: It depends upon movement (exercise) and breath for stimulation. Properly used, the lungs act as sort of a suction pump for the lymphatic system. Combining deep breathing with exercise will do much to improve lymph flow and thus the body's detoxification ability and general state of health. Slow movement exercises such as yoga and tai chi will also work the lymph glands. Yoga, which I like to do, focuses on stretching and controlled breathing. It's empowering to know that something as simple (and free) as breathing can be a powerful tool to build health.

ENERGIZING DOES A BODY GOOD

It comes as no surprise that exercise is an important element in a health-building regimen. It's of course one of the most important things you can do for your overall health. It is also very important in the detoxification process because it stimulates and mobilizes the lymphatic system, which dumps toxins into the circulatory system where they can be processed by the liver and eliminated through the bladder or colon. This action also aids immunity.

The benefits of exercise have long been reported. In addition to its positive impact on the lymphatic system, some of the other benefits include

- increased stamina and energy
- increased flexibility
- increased blood circulation
- better sleep
- stress reduction
- increased self-esteem and sense of well-being
- increased oxygen supply to cells and tissues
- increased muscle strength, tone, and endurance
- release of brain chemicals called endorphins that act as natural tranquilizers
- increased progesterone and decreased estrogen production in women, potentially easing PMS and cramps
- decreased food cravings
- decreased blood sugar levels
- weight distribution and maintenance

Pretty much all of these relate directly to detoxification. Because exercise takes energy from cells, helping them to increase the number and size of the mitochondria (which are your cells' main power generators), you essentially force your cells to work more efficiently and assist with driving toxins out. Moreover, moderate exercise is linked to an improved immune system and an increase in white blood cell activity—both of which positively influence cellular detoxification. Let's not forget how exercise also helps us manage stress better, which can cycle back to boost our immunity further and help us improve our resistance to stress factors that can make us sick and retain more toxins.

One area of exciting study currently under way is how exercise can literally reverse aging. Just last year researchers showed that exercise can help reverse the aging process *at the cellular level.* After six months of resistance training, older participants in the study (whose average age was seventy) exhibited dramatic changes at the genetic level. At the beginning of the six-month period, researchers found significant differences between older and younger participants in the expression of six hundred genes, indicating that these genes become either more or less active with age. By the end of the six months, exercise had changed the expression of a third of

You don't have to join a gym or commit to unrealistic workouts.
Find something you like doing that gets you active.

them—namely those that are involved in the functioning of mitochondria, the powerhouses of cells that process nutrients into energy. This further underscores how exercise can help the detoxification process.

Ideally, a well-rounded and comprehensive exercise program includes cardio work, strength training, and stretching. These three activities each provide unique benefits that your body needs to achieve and maintain peak performance. Today, with so many choices and options for exercise, and a million ways to fit your exercise in even if you have a busy life, there's no excuse for living a sedentary lifestyle. You don't have to join a gym or commit to unrealistic workouts. Find something you like doing that gets you active, whether it's playing volleyball on the beach, going dancing, or hiking in the nearby hills with friends. Plenty of trainers and fitness teachers offer an array of DVDs for rent or sale that you can do in the comfort of home and that will take you step by step through a routine that involves cardio, strength training (sometimes called resistance training), and stretching. Or you can check out that new yoga and spinning studio that just opened up in your neighborhood. It's as simple as that. Get creative and have fun with your activity. Remember, exercise should be enjoyable, something you look forward to every day. Also remember that many forms of exercise can involve your family and friends, which can be very motivating and offer an added benefit.

While your choice of exercise is an individual matter and should reflect your personal preferences, I want to highlight two types of exercise in particular that are especially beneficial for detoxification and that can be enjoyed by virtually everyone, including the elderly and those who may be limited physically and cannot engage in rigorous exercise routines or use standard gym equipment. They are regular walking and the use of a mini trampoline, or "rebounder." These can cover your cardio needs. I'll then share insights on strength training that you can incorporate into your program.

Before You Start

Initiating an exercise program is exciting, and I can't express passionately enough the benefits that await you as you get moving. Just be sure to go at your own pace and please do not jump into any rigorous workout program if you have not been a regular exerciser in the past. The exercises outlined in this chapter are moderate and low-impact, but I know some of you may feel inspired to hop on a StairMaster for hours or start training for a marathon. While I commend those who do get serious with their exercise practices and who do reap enormous, lasting rewards, I want to share a few words of caution. All too often I watch people go too fast and end up tired, strained, and sometimes injured. Before long, they are physically and mentally burned out. They lose interest, and soon enough they are back where they started.

You must achieve a fine balance between pushing your body physically and staying attuned to its needs as you move forward. I strongly recommend speaking with your physician if you have specific health issues or physical limitations to contend with or wish to have guidance in tailoring an exercise program to your physical body. Your doctor can also help you gauge your fitness level so you don't overwork yourself and wind up increasing your risk for injury or illness.

Bear in mind that moderate exercise has profound anti-inflammatory and antistress effects, whereas heavy and prolonged exercise releases huge quantities of stress hormones. For this reason I recommend moderate levels of exercise. Does this mean you shouldn't do an hour of cardio? No. It means that you shouldn't be pushing yourself to complete exhaustion every time you work out. Listen to your body. It will tell you when it's time to stop. Also don't forget that the benefits of exercise are cumulative. You don't have to go at it for a full hour straight. Sprinkle pockets of workout times into your day—at lunch, after dinner, or in the fifteen minutes right after you get up and the house is still quiet.

REBOUNDING TO HEALTH

I encourage rebounding exercises specifically with regard to detoxification because of their simplicity, accessibility, and proven benefits on many fronts. They can also incorporate a jogging or jumping motion, both of which are excellent ways of stimulating blood and lymphatic circulation, helping to move toxins out of their storage sites and out of your body. Most sporting goods stores carry rebounders. You can also go online and find plenty of rebounder suppliers just by Googling "rebounder."

Jogging on a rebounder is easier on your body than jogging on a hard surface. When your feet hit the running surface, there is no resistance—your body is propelled upward and you don't lose energy on the down bounce. When rebounding, on the other hand, there is no risk of injury to your joints. If you are new to the rebounder, you may want to start out with a "soft walk," where you simply shift your weight from one foot to another, lifting your heels as you do so. Even this gentle motion is enough to stimulate lymph flow, helping your body to dissolve and eliminate toxins while strengthening the immune system. Rebounding so effectively moves lymphatic fluid that it has been referred to as "lymphasizing." In addition to clearing the lymph glands, rebounding will provide aerobic exercise (once you've worked up to a sustained motion for fifteen to twenty minutes), oxygenating your body.

When you jump up and down on a rebounder, the force of gravity alternately pulls and then releases each cell, stimulating cellular fluid flow so that toxic material is flushed out and nutrients are absorbed. In addition, the valves in your lymphatic system open and shut when you rebound, pumping lymphatic fluid throughout your body. During this process, not only are toxins removed, but white blood cells are also produced. Even a short (two- to three-minute) rebounding session will dramatically increase your white blood cell production, which has the net effect of increasing immunity. In addition to providing cellular cleansing and enhanced immunity, rebounding exercises the musculoskeletal system, protects and strengthens the cardiovascular and peripheral vascular systems, and helps restore bone density. It is a safe and easy-to-perform exercise for people of any age and in any physical condition. Use your rebounder at least once daily. Short, frequent rebounding sessions can be as beneficial as a single long one.

WALKING OFF THE TOXINS

Walking is one of the most accessible forms of exercise around. You simply put on a good pair of shoes (preferably ones made for walking and/or running) and step outside your front door. It's also the perfect starting point for people who are not accustomed to any type of physical activity. You can go at your own pace and create your own program based on your time and physical shape. For example, schedule twenty- or thirty-minute walks after dinner each night. Or break up those sessions and complete three ten-minute walks throughout your day. Studies now prove that it doesn't matter if you do your workout all at once or in short bursts that add up to the same amount of time spent in a workout each day. You can also add as much or as little intensity to your walks as you like. This is done through speed, inclines and declines, and how long you spend walking.

The simple act of walking pumps lymph nodes, which are concentrated in the neck, underarms, groin, and behind the knees. Again, this helps move toxins out of the body. As you build up to longer, more rigorous walks you'll begin to sweat more and unload toxins through your skin. Walking can be an excellent cardio workout, and you may even advance into the world of power walking if you are so moved. The type of cardio exercise or activity you do is not nearly as important as how you do it, how often you do it, and how long you do it. Keep in mind that cardio is all about increasing the workload of your lungs and heart. It should increase your heart rate and get you breathing rather quickly (and deeply). Leisurely, slow-paced strolls won't do this, though they are a good start.

Start Slowly, Increase Gradually

If you are transitioning from a sedentary lifestyle into one that incorporates regular exercise, start slowly, with a short walk and/or a short session on the rebounder. Gradually increase the time you engage in the activity and the intensity of your effort. If walking, work up to a sustained fast pace for fifteen to twenty minutes. Breathe deeply as you walk, letting your arms swing in a "cross-crawl" motion, so that the right arm is swinging forward at the same time the left foot is put forward—a brisk marching movement.

Remember not to overdo it. You may wish to start with one five-minute rebounder session per day and/or one ten-minute walk daily (or five or six times per week). You would then gradually increase your rebounding or walking time until it is doubled and/or add an extra short rebounder session, as time in your schedule permits. Another option would be to rebound and walk on alternate days. If you have another form of exercise that you prefer, by all means continue doing it. Just consider adding a little rebounding to the mix. The particulars of your program are not nearly as important as your commitment to setting up a routine and goals and sticking with them! If you find yourself working out seven days a week, I encourage you to set aside one day for rest. This will help you to avoid burnout and give your body a much-needed time-out to recover.

EXERCISE BANDS: STRENGTH TRAINING

Another type of exercise that I highly recommend doing in conjunction with your walking and rebounding regimen employs exercise bands. These involve stretching flexible elastic bands or tubes, which provides a progressive stimulus to your muscles to help build lean mass and increase strength. This approach, used initially in rehabilitation settings, is rapidly becoming the rage in a variety of fitness and sports settings. The bands are extremely portable and don't take up much space, fitting easily into your overnight bag or purse. You can go through a complete workout program using just a couple of bands with different resistance levels. You can also recruit ordinary household items such as broom handles, small chairs, or stools to enhance the effect. And you don't need a lot of space to do your routine.

Also, unlike some other forms of exercise, working out with the bands does not aggravate my chronic neck problems. People with pain issues can safely and comfortably work with resistance bands in a number of effective ways. Unlike exercise machines and dumbbells, bands don't rely on the force of gravity to provide resistance. It's the stretching of the band that creates the resistance: the further you stretch it, the greater the resistance. It's that simple!

Regardless of whether you use bands or elect a more traditional approach to strength training, you can expect to experience a number of benefits, including

I use the bands in my daily exercise routine and find that they accommodate my busy lifestyle perfectly, allowing me to work out while traveling without having to locate a gym.

- **Injury prevention through correction of muscle imbalances**

- **Delay (or even reversal) of muscle mass loss experienced with aging**

- **Decrease in total cholesterol and improvement in the ratio of good to bad cholesterol (lowering the risk of heart disease)**

- **Increased bone density**

- **Increased circulation that moves toxins and amplifies the body's detox processes**

A single band can be used to perform a multitude of exercises that will strengthen every major muscle group in your body. It can even work on some muscles, such as the rotator cuff over the shoulder joint, that machines don't impact. The cost of setting up such a tubing gym is amazingly low: under $75. You can get by on much less, however, because you can get a lot of mileage out of a single band, with an investment of less than $5! Your home becomes your gym without the need for any major modifications or additions to the contents. The freedom of motion offered by these bands is inherent in the fact they can be adjusted to accommodate body size and shape and used in virtually any position. With the aid of resistance bands, you can exercise all muscle groups, including the smaller ones. By strengthening these, you help prevent injury.

The bands don't just increase strength—they help build flexibility, power, balance, and speed. And because they improve circulation, they stimulate cellular fluid flow to move toxins, as well as give your lymphatic system a boost. The net result is that these simple, lightweight, inexpensive rubber resistance bands can help you maximize your body's detoxification at the cellular level (not to mention burn off fat, which releases toxins, while increasing lean muscle mass and improving your overall fitness).

You can purchase exercise resistance bands at many fitness and sporting goods stores, as well as online (see the Resource Directory for leads). Most bands will come with instructions and a basic program for you to follow. In my last book, *The Fiber35 Diet: Nature's Weight Loss Secret,* I outlined a complete strength training routine using the bands, which includes both upper and lower body workouts. You can now download this program at www.detoxstrategy.com. There you will also find tips to using a rebounder and scheduling these two types of exercise into your week.

In addition to the use of resistance bands, strength training can also be achieved through other practices, chiefly Pilates and certain forms of yoga such as Ashtanga or Vinyasa flow. These practices engage multiple muscles (often with the body's own weight as resistance), increase circulation, and demand core strength. They also enhance flexibility, balance, coordination, and posture—all excellent goals for vibrant health. The core can be one of the more difficult areas to work, but strengthening the core is vital to maintaining good physical conditioning. It even can improve digestion; a fit core with strong lower abdominal muscles has been proven to aid in the health of the digestive system. This ultimately assists the detoxification process overall. Both yoga and Pilates are best done with the help of an instructor at a studio or gym, especially if you are a beginner. A class setting will also encourage proper form and teach you the poses. Pilates can entail the use of machines or can be performed on a mat. One of my favorite brands of Pilates is called Polestar Pilates. You may want to check out their website at www.PolestarPilates.com to see if there is a center or studio near you.

Stretching and Cooling Down

Don't forget to stretch *after* any exercise routine (never before). Stretching is important to keep your body limber, but it should not be done without having warmed up your muscles first through other exercises. Once used, the muscles will be easier to stretch due to the fact they have a higher core temperature and thus a greater blood—and lymph—flow. By stretching a fatigued muscle, you help it recover faster, prevent tightening, and increase flexibility. You'll get maximal benefit out of each stretch by holding it for 30 to 60 seconds.

Try to incorporate stretching into your cool-down period following your workout session. This is when your body functions are stabilizing— your previously elevated heart rate is normalizing and you stop perspiring. During this period of time, you'll want to drink some water and relax in a quiet environment, while gently stretching your fatigued muscles, one group at a time.

MIND YOUR SPIRIT

Exercise is not always about strenuous movement and sweating it out on a treadmill or long walk. Sometimes we need to exercise more than our physical bodies by addressing and nurturing that all-important mind-body connection. Just as science has proven time and time again the benefits of exercise, so it has with relaxation and stress-reduction techniques.

I'm a big believer in engaging in activities that help one cope with inevitable stress. We all live busy lives and typically have more to-dos that we can possibly handle. One of the most amazing benefits of relaxation is that it can give you an inner peace, which then translates to a multitude of other payoffs. Every area of your life will get better. You'll enjoy increased confidence and a sense of well-being. You'll get more accomplished both at work and home during the day. Your body will feel more alive and able to tackle minor illnesses like colds and flus. And you'll find it easier to navigate through stressful periods. Maintaining a relaxed mind will also help you to sleep better at night, which is sadly becoming one of the hardest things for people to do lately. Sleep is so critical to overall health and wellness, though, that without high-quality hours of this magical ingredient banked in your busy body, you won't be able to reap all the benefits that this program has to offer. Neither will you be able to rejuvenate and renew your body at the cellular level.

For some people, physical exercise is enough to accomplish the task of destressing and relaxing. But for others, practices such as yoga and meditation are more effective. I take yoga classes as well as practice meditation routinely. I find that these truly help me to relax and manage stress, become more attuned to my body and its needs, and tap a source of renewed strength and spirit to deal with whatever stressful factors come my way.

Experiment with a few relaxation techniques to find what works best for you (unless you already know). If classes are not accessible to you, plenty of videos and DVDs are on the market for taking you through classic yoga and meditation sessions at every level. Remember, the practice of deep breathing itself can afford you tremendous benefits. It can be enough to stimulate your body's intrinsic detoxifying processes via the movement of lymph. Here's how you do it: Place your hands along your rib cage at the level of your sternum. As you inhale, you should feel your belly and ribs expanding, and then as you exhale, you'll feel them collapsing. Try practicing four to six long breaths—inhaling for six counts, and exhaling for six counts. Aim to do this exercise two or three times a day (it can be done anywhere, even at a desk or on the couch in front of the TV). You'll notice a lift in your attitude and a decline in your stress.

Stress management can also come in the form of counseling and reading enlightening material, which can help reframe our interpretation of stressful events so that they will have less of an impact on our emotions, thus mitigating the release of the stress hormones, which can then enhance the detox processes.

A relaxed body and mind is a more efficiently operating mind and body. In fact, meditation has been shown to be associated with structural changes in the brain that may slow down the aging-related atrophy of certain areas of the brain. In other words, meditation not only helps you cope better with stress, but it may also help you keep your brain young and functioning optimally.

If you are under a lot of stress on a regular basis and find yourself routinely lacking energy, you may want to consider adding a nutritional supplement designed specifically to aid your adrenal glands so they can handle the load. Stress hormones such as cortisol can run amok and impair not only your metabolism but the workings of your overall bodily systems in general. For this reason I recommend looking for an adrenal support supplement formula. Key ingredients include the B vitamin pantothenic acid, the amino acid L-theanine, and extracts of banaba, *Rhodiola rosea,* ashwagandha, and eleuthero root (a form of ginseng).

SLEEP TIGHT

Our knowledge about the power of sleep has gained more clarity in recent years. A new public interest in sleep ignited in late 2004 when scientists demonstrated a strong connection between one's sleep patterns and ability to lose weight, which ignited a new public interest in sleep. Since then, sleep research continues to provide fascinating insights into the power of sleep in the support of health and longevity. Just about every system in the body, including the detoxification process, is affected by the quality and amount of sleep you get a night.

One aspect to sleep that is especially influential to our overall health and general sense of well-being is its control of our hormonal cycles. A healthy day/night cycle is tied into our normal hormonal secretion patterns—from those associated with our eating patterns to those that relate to stress and cellular recovery. Cortisol, for example, should be highest in the morning and progressively decrease throughout the day, with the lowest levels occurring after 11 P.M. With low evening cortisol levels, melatonin levels rise. Melatonin is your body's natural hormone that tells you it's time to sleep. Higher melatonin levels will allow for more REM (rapid eye movement) sleep, which helps maintain healthy levels of growth hormone, thyroid hormone, and male and female sex hormones. In fact, growth hormone gets released mostly at night when you're filling your sleep bank with quality, restful sleep. This is the hormone necessary for cellular repair and rejuvenation. If you miss out on deep sleep, not only will you feel sluggish and nonrefreshed the next day, but your body will have missed out on getting its much-needed levels of growth hormone.

I understand that sleep can be difficult to get today in our 24/7 lives, but make it a goal to do what you can to sleep at least eight hours a night. It helps to wind down thirty minutes to an hour before bedtime and prepare for sleep by taking a warm bath, light reading, or having a cup of herbal tea such as chamomile or lavender. Getting a full eight hours is critical to maintaining your metabolism, which then directly affects the strength of your body's detoxification. I know that this much time may require you to sacrifice late-night television or surfing the Internet, but if you choose sleep, you'll effectively amplify your detox program and accelerate your journey down this path to wellness.

Chapter 7 Summary

- Exercise imparts numerous benefits, including helping to detoxify the body through increased circulation, deep breathing, sweating, and stimulating the lymphatic system. The role of the lymphatic system is to gather toxins.

- It's important to find an activity that you like and that gets your body moving. It can be moderate and if you have not exercised in a while you can begin with low-impact walking. Start slowly and increase gradually. Exercise is cumulative, so you don't have to do it all at once.

- You can get a complete workout that enhances your natural detoxification system through several simple types of exercise:

    - walking
    - rebounding
    - using resistance bands
    - core strength exercises such as Pilates and yoga

- Finding ways to relax and cope with stress is critical to maintaining your health and encouraging detoxification. If you're constantly under a lot of stress, you may want to supplement your diet with an adrenal support formula.

- Getting a good night's sleep is vital to health. Shoot for eight hours a night.

CHAPTER 8

STEP FIVE: WELLNESS (PUTTING IT ALL TOGETHER)

❧

Congratulations. If you have arrived at this last step and already applied some of the recommendations given in this book to your life, you are on your way to being in the best health that you can be. The last step in the RENEW program is really the part when you see the entire plan in action. It's your daily schedule that will keep you on the path to optimum wellness.

❧

Step 5 is about putting together and following a personal schedule that works with your life. Everyone must set forth his or her own personal plan for jump-starting, nurturing, and maintaining that W: Wellness. This entails not only the daily decisions you make, but also the weekly, monthly, and yearly actions you take to continue supporting your all-important W.

Fostering a healthy body is not something you can do through a single action. It requires a commitment to constant vigilance in your environment, honoring your dietary changes regularly, as well as completing periodically procedures such as colon hydrotherapy or total-body basic cleanses every six months. Remember, the essence of the RENEW program is simply a blueprint consisting of practical concepts and easy, actionable steps that can help you achieve a more vibrant, healthier you—a you that will be able to sustain the perils of living in a polluted world, as well as the (often) unavoidable hazards related to aging. It's a multisystem approach for total-body health and transformation.

You will look better, sleep more soundly, have fewer aches and pains.

No matter what your primary goals are for cleaning up your environment and aiding in the natural detoxification of your body, one truth is certain: you will likely achieve results you never thought possible. You will not only feel better generally and welcome brighter, more vibrant health, but you will *look* better, sleep more soundly, have fewer aches and pains, and rank your overall sense of well-being much higher than ever before. If you are looking to lose weight or simply maintain your current weight, this detoxification program will assist you in that endeavor. Anyone who carries around excess weight will likely see pounds drop off through this program *even if you don't make a concerted effort to lose weight* using a strict diet and/or rigorous exercise regimen. The nature of this RENEW program will essentially reboot your body and help it return to a more natural state where it enjoys its own unique, ideal weight.

As you have already learned, once pathogens and toxins have entered the bloodstream, they are carried first to the liver and then on to other organs throughout the body. If the liver's detoxification ability is impaired due to nutritional deficiency and/or toxic overload, these toxins will be stored (often in the weakest areas of the body such as fat) and can initiate chronic disease.

Eliminating sickness from the body entails two simultaneous steps: one is to evict the main cause of the ailment and the other is to elevate the body's general vitality so that its natural and inherent ability to sustain health is allowed to dominate. Granted, sometimes we can't always remove the culprit at the root of our sickness, which can be an unknown in many cases. But we can do what we can to take as much control of our bodies as possible to balance their functions and boost the immune system. And to do this, we start by detoxifying the body at the cellular level. Hopefully, by now you also have made plans to clean up your environment to limit and manage the very toxins that continue to undermine your systems of health. Now it's time to see how the RENEW strategy comes together in a daily schedule, and establish its main tenets as a way of life.

SAMPLE CLEANSING AND DETOX SCHEDULES

The following are sample schedules to give you an idea on how to incorporate all the elements of the program. You may wish to alter them to suit your individual times and needs. You may substitute a protein drink for the morning or afternoon snack if you feel you need more protein. Choose a whole-food multinutrient from pea and rice protein if you are vegetarian, as described in Chapter 6. (See Chapter 11 for protein recipes.) You can also have a cup of herbal tea before bedtime—chamomile or lavender is nice and relaxing. For your bedtime fiber supplement, choose one that is organic and contains good sources of fiber such as flax, acacia, and gluten-free oat bran. Although some people choose psyllium as their fiber supplement, for many this type of fiber can be dehydrating to the colon, contributing to a more constipated state. You simply want a supplement that you can take easily with water (not a shake or bar that could be too heavy before bedtime). Refer back to Chapter 5 for the basic outlines, aims, and components of the cleansing programs. Also don't forget to go to www.detoxstrategy.com for additional support and resources.

Throughout the day, make sure you are consuming at least eight glasses of water daily, up to half your body weight in ounces. You may freely drink vegetable broth throughout the day, which will count as water intake. You can schedule colon hydrotherapy sessions during the week per your therapist's guidance and advice.

Total-Body BASIC
Cleanse Schedule

6:00 A.M.   Wake up. Drink glass of room-temperature or warm fresh-squeezed lemon water. Take one dose of probiotic supplement.

6:30 A.M.   10 to 20 minutes of exercise—rebounding, bands, yoga, or cardio. Drink a glass of water during or after exercise.

7:00 A.M.   Take morning dose of total-body basic herbal detox product with glass of water. Dry skin brush whole body before showering.

7:30 A.M.   Have a good breakfast.* Choose from breakfast choices in Chapter 11. Take enzymes, oils, and a whole-food multinutrient with the meal.

10:30 A.M.   Have a fiber drink. Choose from fiber choices in Chapter 11.

11:00 A.M.   Have 1 ounce liquid greens supplement with 8 ounces of water, glass of fresh vegetable juice, or cup of broth.

12:30 P.M.   Have lunch.* Choose from lunch recipes in Chapter 11. Take enzymes with meal.

2:00 P.M.   Have a fiber drink. Choose from fiber choices in Chapter 11.

3:00 P.M.   Have 1 ounce liquid greens supplement with 8 ounces of water, glass of fresh vegetable juice, or cup of broth.

5:00 P.M.   Optional short rebounding session (5 to 10 minutes).

6:00 P.M.   Have dinner.* Choose from dinner recipes in Chapter 11. Take enzymes and oils with meal.

7:00 P.M.   Optional walk for 15 or 20 minutes.

8:00 P.M.   Sauna or soak. Relax and meditate.

9:00 P.M.   Take evening dose of total-body basic herbal detox product and fiber supplement before bed with glass of water. Optional: herbal tea.

*For those who choose to do a three-day fast at the start of the detox, you will substitute your meals with a freshly made juice drink (choose from juice recipes in Chapter 11). The vegetable broth can be consumed throughout the day. Make sure to drink plenty of water during the day.

TOTAL-BODY **ADVANCED**
CLEANSE SCHEDULE

6:00 A.M.   Wake up. Drink glass of room-temperature or warm fresh-squeezed lemon water. Take one dose of probiotic supplement.

6:30 A.M.   10 to 20 minutes of exercise—rebounding, bands, yoga, or cardio. Drink a glass of water during or after exercise.

7:00 A.M.   Take morning dose of total-body advanced herbal detox product with glass of water. Dry skin brush whole body before showering.

7:30 A.M.   Have a good breakfast. Choose from breakfast choices in Chapter 11. Take enzymes, oils, and a whole-food multinutrient with the meal.

10:30 A.M.   Have a fiber drink. Choose from fiber choices in Chapter 11.

11:00 A.M.   Have 1 ounce liquid greens supplement with 8 ounces of water, glass of fresh vegetable juice, or cup of broth.

12:30 P.M.   Have lunch. Choose from lunch recipes in Chapter 11. Take enzymes with meal.

2:00 P.M.   Have a fiber drink. Choose from fiber choices in Chapter 11.

3:00 P.M.   Have 1 ounce liquid greens supplement with 8 ounces of water, glass of fresh vegetable juice, or cup of broth.

5:00 P.M.   Optional short rebounding session (5 to 10 minutes).

6:00 P.M.   Have dinner. Choose from dinner recipes in Chapter 11. Take enzymes and oils with meal.

7:00 P.M.   Optional walk for 15 or 20 minutes.

8:00 P.M.   Sauna or soak. Relax and meditate.

9:00 P.M.   Take evening dose of total-body advanced herbal detox product and fiber supplement before bed with glass of water.

Targeted LIVER
Cleanse Schedule

6:00 A.M.	Wake up. Drink glass of room-temperature or warm fresh-squeezed lemon water. Take one dose of probiotic supplement.
6:30 A.M.	10 to 20 minutes of exercise—rebounding, bands, yoga, or cardio. Drink a glass of water during or after exercise.
7:00 A.M.	Take morning dose of liver cleanse detox formula with glass of water. Dry skin brush whole body before showering.
7:30 A.M.	Have a good breakfast. Choose from breakfast choices in Chapter 11. Take enzymes, oils, and a whole-food multinutrient with the meal.
10:30 A.M.	Have a fiber drink. Choose from fiber choices in Chapter 11.
11:00 A.M.	Have 1 ounce liquid greens supplement with 8 ounces of water, glass of fresh vegetable juice, or cup of broth.
12:30 P.M.	Have lunch. Choose from lunch recipes in Chapter 11. Take enzymes with meal.
2:00 P.M.	Have a fiber drink. Choose from fiber choices in Chapter 11.
3:00 P.M.	Have 1 ounce liquid greens supplement with 8 ounces of water, glass of fresh vegetable juice, or cup of broth.
5:00 P.M.	Optional short rebounding session (5 to 10 minutes).
6:00 P.M.	Have dinner. Choose from dinner recipes in Chapter 11. Take enzymes and oils with meal.
7:00 P.M.	Optional walk for 15 or 20 minutes.
8:00 P.M.	Sauna or soak. Relax and meditate.
9:00 P.M.	Take evening dose of liver cleanse herbal detox product and fiber supplement before bed with glass of water.

TARGETED HEAVY METAL
CLEANSE SCHEDULE

6:00 A.M.	Wake up. Drink glass of room-temperature or warm fresh-squeezed lemon water. Take one dose of probiotic supplement.
6:30 A.M.	10 to 20 minutes of exercise—rebounding, bands, yoga, or cardio. Drink a glass of water during or after exercise.
7:00 A.M.	Dry skin brush whole body before showering.
7:30 A.M.	Have a good breakfast. Choose from breakfast choices in Chapter 11. Take enzymes, oils, and a whole-food multinutrient with the meal. Take morning dose of heavy metal cleanse herbal detox product with glass of water at breakfast.
10:30 A.M	Have a fiber drink. Choose from fiber choices in Chapter 11.
11:00 A.M.	Have 1 ounce liquid greens supplement with 8 ounces of water, glass of fresh vegetable juice, or cup of broth.
12:30 P.M.	Have lunch. Choose from lunch recipes in Chapter 11. Take enzymes with meal.
2:00 P.M.	Have a fiber drink. Choose from fiber choices in Chapter 11.
3:00 P.M.	Have 1 ounce liquid greens supplement with 8 ounces of water, glass of fresh vegetable juice, or cup of broth.
5:00 P.M.	Take evening dose of heavy metal cleanse herbal detox product with a glass of water.
5:30 P.M.	Optional short rebounding session (5 to 10 minutes).
6:00 P.M.	Have dinner. Choose from dinner recipes in Chapter 11. Take enzymes and oils with meal.
7:00 P.M.	Optional walk for 15 or 20 minutes.
8:00 P.M.	Sauna or soak. Relax and meditate.
9:00 P.M.	Take fiber supplement before bed with glass of water.

HEALTH MAINTENANCE SUPPLEMENTS AND REMINDERS

Following is an outline of supplements and suggestions to recap the ideas of RENEW and help you maintain your newfound health.

Daily Doses of Support

Following is a list of supplements to consider on a daily basis, depending on your particular circumstances. They will help support the natural structure and functions of your body and encourage a healthy self-detoxification system.

Supplements Highly Recommended for Everyone

- multivitamin and mineral formula
- omega-3 fatty acids (fish oil)
- calcium and magnesium (for women)
- magnesium (for men)
- fiber
- probiotics

Optional Supplements as Needed

- digestive enzymes
- amino acids
- whole-food multinutrient
- liquid greens

Weekly Commitments

- Exercise at least four to five days a week.

- Take saunas and steambaths two to three times per week or as often as your health care professional recommends, working within the limits of your time constraints and financial considerations.

Annual Cleansings

- two-step herbal cleansing at least twice a year

- targeted herbal programs once a year

- hydrotherapy, based on your colon hydrotherapist's advice

In the Resource Directory you'll find a list of cleansing and detoxification centers across the United States. Some of these allow for weekly stays, which can be especially helpful to those dealing with multiple health issues or who simply need more structure.

TOXIC MYTHS AND THE TRAIL OF CHEMICALS IN OUR DAILY LIVES

❧

The ubiquity of pollutants in our bodies was recently brought to the attention of Canadian politicians, and reported with the comedic heading "Pollutants in Politics: Chemical Testing Reveals Party Leaders' Toxic Relationship." But it was no laughing matter. When leaders of Ontario's three main parties voluntarily gave blood and urine samples to environmentalists to be analyzed for seventy chemical contaminants linked to health problems, all three carried a bewildering variety of pesticides, residues from stain and grease repellents, and compounds used in plastics.

❧

In addition to testing positive for high levels of bisphenol A, a chemical that mimics the female sex hormone estrogen and is used to make consumer products ranging from plastic baby bottles to the linings of tin cans, the politicians were also tested for polychlorinated biphenyls, chemicals used in electrical transformers that were banned decades ago. Despite no longer being in use, PCBs are so persistent that all the politicians tested positive for them. The highest chemical exposures they had? Phthalates (pronounced *thal*-ates), a class of chemicals used to soften plastic and a primary component of the polyvinyl chloride in cars that gives off that "new car smell" from the interior.

Phthalates are also used as gelling agents and fixatives in cosmetics and grooming products; they are what make drug capsules soft and baby books for bathtubs squishy. If you recall that tangy taste of water from a hose, that's the phthalates used to give the plastic in the hose its flexibility. The article was quick to point out the fact that male politicians are exposed more than most men to these toxins because they typically have makeup applied before appearing in television studios. What if the politicians were women who wear makeup every day? Male fetuses exposed to phthalates in the womb may result in malformation of the reproductive tract and decreased semen quality later in life.

It would be impossible to cover every toxin and its related effects in this book. Doing justice to just the most common toxins we encounter today would require hundreds of pages. So what we're going to do is look at a handful of toxins that virtually all of us typically meet routinely in our daily lives—but probably don't even know it. They arise from air, water, food, and household products, many of which come from unlikely places. We'll start by looking at an average person's everyday habits, which will reinforce the need to detoxify and further help clarify where these chemicals lurk persistently.

A DAY IN THE LIFE

Ever wondered if you would pass an FDA inspection?

7:00 A.M. Good morning. You wake up in a cozy bed that's made with several ingredients that your body absorbs during the night, including toluene (a chemical linked to birth defects and emitted from the polyurethane foam that makes your bed so comfy), a stain-resistant chemical called perfluorooctanoic acid, fire-retardant chemicals linked to learning disorders and thyroid dysfunction, and antimony, an element linked to heart and lung problems. As of July 1, 2007, all mattresses manufactured or imported into the United States must be treated with these fire-retardant chemicals. After you rise out of bed, you lumber to the bathroom across your synthetic carpet that's also full of chemicals to keep it stainless and less likely to combust in a house fire.

7:05 A.M. Now you're brushing your teeth with toothpaste that comes with a warning label that reads something like this: *Keep out of reach of children under 6 years of age. If more than used for brushing is accidentally swallowed, get medical help or contact Poison Control Center right away.* This label exists because you are exposed to sodium fluoride, linked to enzyme disruption and thyroid problems; sodium lauryl sulfate, linked to organ and reproductive toxicity; triclosan, an antibacterial agent that's registered as a pesticide with the EPA, and which is linked to organ toxicity and possibly cancer. If you finished up your dental hygiene with a gargle of mouthwash, which also comes with a warning label, you taste more than its active ingredients. It may contain formaldehyde and ammonia in addition to several flavoring and coloring chemicals, as well as some chemicals that have leached from the plastic in the bottle.

7:15 A.M. Take a shower. Depending on your water source and the use of filters, you could be exposing yourself to chlorine, fluoride, lead, copper, alpha emitters (elements such as radon, uranium, and radium, all of which are linked to cancer), and trihalomethanes, by-products produced from adding chlorine to disinfect the water. Trihalomethanes are linked to bladder and colorectal cancer, and exposure through drinking and skin absorption has been shown in studies to increase one's chance of miscarriages and other reproductive problems. Haloacetic acids may also be present in your water, which are also by-products of chlorine's disinfection, and are classified by the EPA as possible cancer-causing agents. In addition, traces of herbicides and pharmaceutical drugs may also be present. Tap water is not as clean as the government would like us to think. (I'll explain how drugs get into your tap water a bit later.)

Depending on the type of soap and shampoo you use, you expose yourself to coloring agents, dyes, artificial preservatives, and propylene glycol, a lubricant and suspected carcinogen.

7:30 A.M. Apply antiperspirant to "keep you dry" during your hectic day. Most contain aluminum zirconium, which is toxic to the nervous and reproductive systems, a chemical called BHT, which is believed to be a hormonal disrupter and neurotoxin, and various chemicals that give your deodorant stick that distinctive smell. You'll also get another dose of propylene glycol, which helps the deodorant go on so nicely but is linked to irritation and immune toxicity.

7:35 A.M. Time to get dressed. You pull up pants or slip on a dress that just came back from the dry cleaner. Now the garments carry a litany of chemical fumes and residues including perchloroethylene, also known as perc tetrachloroethylene, PCE, perclene, and perchlor. This chemical is believed to be capable of causing cancer, especially in the liver and kidneys. It is also shown to effect developing fetuses. If you think you're safe because your clothes are not dry-cleaned, are they 100 percent natural? Or do you have synthetic fibers (think polyester) in your clothing? If so, they may be off-gassing (sometimes called outgassing, which is releasing or giving off as a gas or vapor) small molecules of plasticizer fumes, plus flame-retardant chemicals. Got mothballs in your closet? Those can deliver an unhealthy dose of the carcinogenic pesticide dichlorobenzene (also found in toilet deodorizers). And if you're getting dressed in the confines of a walk-in closet or a well-insulated bedroom, you are increasing the concentration of these chemical gases emitting from your clothes. Let's not forget other nearby sources of invisible gases, like those from your carpet, rugs, painted walls, and furniture.

FACT

A group of compounds called endocrine disrupters are getting a lot of attention as infertility rates skyrocket and more and more *young* women complain of having trouble conceiving and giving birth to healthy children. Endocrine disrupters mimic or block hormones that regulate many bodily functions, such as estrogen, progesterone, and testosterone—hormones that are key to reproductive health. Small changes to this intricate system of hormonal signals can translate to major health concerns that could be difficult, if not impossible, to reverse.

Perc Is No Perk

In early 2007, California regulators enacted the nation's first statewide ban on the most common chemical used by dry cleaners. By 2023, no more dry-cleaning machines that use the toxic solvent perchloroethylene ("perc") will be permitted in the state. California declared perc a toxic chemical in 1991. State health officials agree that it can cause lymphoma and cancers of the esophagus, cervix, and bladder.

7:45 A.M. As you apply makeup—foundation, blush, mascara, lipstick, and so on—you are exposed to parabens, which are believed to cause breast cancer and birth abnormalities; artificial colorants, which are suspected carcinogens toxic to the nervous system; triethanolamine, which is linked to cancer, allergies, and immune toxicity; and BHA, a chemical that may cause cancer, hormonal imbalances, and be toxic to organs and the immune system. If you apply body lotion, you likely use the kind that contains chemicals to aid in its skin penetration, which can also push toxins from your other cosmetics deeper into your skin.

MYTH

The government would not let us be exposed to anything harmful.

7:55 A.M. Here comes the hair spray, which probably smells toxic, because it is. Its ingredients can affect your nervous, reproductive, and immune systems. Hair gels, mousses, and cream conditioners are equally toxic.

8:00 A.M. Have you had your first cup of coffee yet? Or maybe you prefer the buzz from a diet soda, again loaded with chemicals and artificial sweeteners. While caffeine does afford people some benefits, including a temporary boost of energy, too much can result in a cycle of highs and lows that can ultimately wreak havoc on steady levels of energy-promoting and detoxing hormones. Additionally, caffeine can increase the rate at which you lose nutrients, which can aggravate your condition by taking away your body's supply of the very nutrients it needs for proper detoxification.

8:15 A.M. You pour yourself some cereal with milk. It's likely laced with food additives and preservatives, including an artificial sweetener linked to all kinds of health problems, from allergies to behavior problems, brain tumors, neurological diseases, and cancer. As you multitask in the kitchen, you make yourself a sandwich for lunch, again with foods loaded with additives and preservatives including nitrates, antibiotics, and synthetic hormones. You then wrap it in plastic that contains vinyl chloride, known to cause cancer in the brain, liver, and lungs. You load up the dishwasher and turn it on before you go, but not before you get a good whiff of the chlorine in its first washing stage. Of course, all those cleaning chemicals lying underneath your sink are also emitting unnoticeable fumes into the air you breathe.

8:30 A.M. Don't you love the smell of that new car? On your way to work you sit in a sea of gases coming from the plastics, fabrics, solvents, and glues in your car. These include polyvinyl chloride, xylene, styrene, and ethylbenzene. If you open your window to let in the fresh air, you inhale the fumes from the cars around you. (The off-gassing of chemicals from a new car can take months or years to go away. A 2003 study in Japan found that the chemicals present in a new minivan were more than 35 times the health limit. In four months they had fallen under the limit but increased again in the hot summer months, taking three years to remain permanently below the limit.)

All this before 9:00 in the morning! The list continues throughout your day as you work under fluorescent lighting, lunch at a fast food restaurant, and take in all the gases floating around your breathing spaces.

A DOSE OF REALITY

Before you pack up the car and think about living off the land in a remote corner of the country, let's get one thing straight. We may live in a toxic soup but we can't escape it by moving to a far-off location, pretending it's not there, or redefining what "normal" is. You can't seek safety even in the Arctic Circle; the by-products and chemicals from our civilizations to the south have landed in this pristine area of the world via air currents. Dust particles grab onto toxic chemicals and travel north to colder climates, which explains why animals and humans who live in the most desolate patches of the globe—thousands of miles from sources of pollution—are showing signs of significant contamination. Inuit women carry toxic levels of PCBs, such that their breast milk would be deemed hazardous by FDA standards.

If the above litany of toxins surprises you, let's consider some of the biggest myths out there with regard to toxins.

As we saw in Chapter 1, it's impossible to know exactly how many synthetic chemicals exist in the world today. And, according to toxins expert Dr. Doris Rapp, the "rules" have been written in such a way that we can never know what is safe until people or wildlife begin suffering. A tremendous amount of politicking is involved with the passage of regulatory laws on the one hand, and chemical manufacturing on the other. Originally, Congress passed the Toxic Substances Control Act (TSCA) in 1976 as a means of giving the Environmental Protection Agency (EPA) a way to track industrial chemicals produced within or imported into the United States, and to be a means for the federal government to require comprehensive health and safety testing for all new and existing chemicals.

But now the TSCA is one of the weakest environmental laws in the United States. The Chemical Manufacturers Association has waged a fierce battle against this act, mainly because of the safety testing requirements. Contrary to its original intent, the TSCA rule is exclusive of mandatory health and safety testing on chemicals. Instead, through the TSCA, the EPA can require safety testing only if they can prove that the chemical poses an unreasonable risk of injury to health or the environment.

This may not sound so hard to do, but it is, because the same law basically prohibits the EPA from mandating health studies from the Chemical Manufacturers Association. In other words, the only safety testing done is by the chemical manufacturers themselves—which many have said is like having the fox guarding the henhouse!

In 1990 the Organization for Economic Cooperation and Development

(OECD), through the initiative of Dr. John Moore, who served as acting administrator of the EPA, initiated a voluntary testing program for High Production Volume (HPV) chemicals. To show their cooperation the Chemical Manufacturers Association agreed to "conditional" support of the testing program. The conditions and criteria set by the CMA led to long delays upon implementation of the program, including a screening program for chemicals that would identify the ones that may need actual testing. In other words, they again stated that the OECD, like the EPA in the 1976 Act, had to show that a chemical may do harm and need safety testing. To date the list of OECD High Production Volume chemicals includes 4,843 substances, with an estimated 7 percent having had the suggested safety testing.

It's naive to assume that all chemicals introduced into our environment or used in marketed products would have at the very least basic safety testing performed before we were exposed to them. Even the EPA states that this "is not a prudent assumption." Consider the story of the now infamous DDT as a case in point. DDT is one of the best-known synthetic pesticides of the modern era. This chlorine-based chemical was first synthesized in 1874 but its insecticidal properties were not discovered until 1939. In the early years of World War II, it combated mosquitoes spreading malaria, typhus, and other insect-borne human diseases among both military and civilian populations. The Swiss chemist Paul Hermann Müller of Geigy Pharmaceutical (now Ciba-Geigy) was awarded the Nobel Prize in Physiology or Medicine in 1948 "for his discovery of the high efficiency of DDT as a contact poison against several arthropods." After the war, DDT's production skyrocketed as it made its way into the agricultural world, where it was used as a potent insecticide.

But with all the focus on how powerful and effective DDT was on insects, no one focused on its health consequences to not only human life but other animal life. Sadly, with no safety testing done prior to its widespread use, it affected and harmed millions of unsuspecting humans and wildlife, especially birds. When Rachel Carson's groundbreaking *Silent Spring* was published in 1962, which cataloged the environmental impacts of the indiscriminate spraying of DDT in the United States and questioned the logic of releasing large amounts of chemicals into the environment without fully understanding their effects on ecology or human health, people began to wonder. Carson suggested that DDT and other pesticides may cause cancer and that their agricultural use was a threat to wildlife. The public outcry that followed eventually led to a ban on DDT for agricultural use (the United States banned it in 1972 for its cancer-causing potential in humans; it also has ties to cardiovascular disease). Today scientists partly attribute the comeback of the bald eagle to this ban. It still may persist in the environment, and though it's no longer used in the United States, it is still produced here and exported to other countries, many of which import the DDT-treated food back to us!

We may have banned DDT, but there are numerous other pesticides in use today that may pose the same risks. In California alone, where nearly one of every four pounds of pesticides is applied in agriculture, forty pesticides are listed as known to cause cancer in animals. But pesticide exposure is not confined to agricultural areas. In urban locations pesticides are used in homes, yards, public buildings, stores, schools, parks, and other settings, resulting in per-acre pesticide intensity in some urban areas that exceeds agricultural use. In the United States a mixture of pesticide residues are detected in the blood and urine of nearly 100 percent of all persons sampled. (For more about pesticides, refer to Appendix A.)

MYTH

Labels tell the whole story.

As absurd as this may sound, companies are not legally required to list all of their ingredients due to trade secrecy laws. In fact, up to 99 percent of ingredients in any product can be withheld from a label if they are categorized as "inert" or "other"—even if they are toxic, pollutants, and hazardous to human health. Some experts have said that the number of hazardous "inert" chemicals totals more than 650 in pesticide products alone, including commonly used bug sprays and insect repellents that may appear at your next picnic.

A total of about 2,500 substances is added to products without you having a clue as to what those substances are or how they could potentially harm you and your family. Vinyl chloride was once considered an "inert" ingredient found in aerosol products such as hair spray and deodorant. If you were to flash back to the early 1970s and get a whiff of the air in hair salons, you'd be inhaling this insidious chemical. When a wave of cancers surfaced in the people who worked at the chemical plants making vinyl chloride, manufacturers rethought this dangerous ingredient and stopped using it for hair spray. Most of today's nail salons smell toxic due to the high concentration of volatile organic compounds (VOCs) filling the air from all those nail care products. The nail industry is not regulated, but the EPA is encouraging salons to convert their toxic products to eco- and people-friendly ones as increasing studies about the effects of long-term exposure to VOCs in nail care products emerge. California is the first state to pass a law that requires cosmetics companies to list all ingredients that can cause cancer and reproductive harm (even if they are deemed "inert"). Hopefully other states will follow.

FACT

When *Time* magazine featured the "Worst Jobs in America" in 2007, topping the list were industrial laundry and dry-cleaning workers because they deal with biohazardous materials and toxic waste on a daily basis. Nail salon workers took the number three spot, also due to their constant exposure to noxious products.

Most people assume that you need to have been exposed to a large dose of toxins in order for any health implications to occur. This is simply not true. Chronic long-term exposure to even the smallest amount of certain toxins can be harmful to your health. For example, the solvent benzene, which increases the risk of leukemia even at small amounts of exposure, is part of our everyday lives. We are regularly exposed to benzene while breathing tobacco smoke, even secondhand smoke, pumping gasoline, while driving in high-traffic areas, and from industrial air pollution. Higher levels are released from the vapors of benzene-containing products such as glues, paints, furniture wax, and detergents. An estimated 44,240 new cases of leukemia will be diagnosed in the United States in 2007. Sometimes chronic low doses can be even *more* toxic than acute high doses. This looks to be especially true when it comes to the toxins that affect your hormonal, or endocrine, system.

MYTH

Toxins are harmless in small amounts.

Moreover, toxic chemicals can react in unexpected ways, especially when combined with other chemicals. Scientists simply cannot predict who is vulnerable to which substances or at which dosages. No one can tell you, for instance, that your body can tolerate chemical A but not chemical B—or that your body can handle x amount of a certain chemical but no more. The factors that trigger illness or disease in any given person are vague and unknown. Whether you are exposed to a few toxic substances or a broad range of synthetics, there's no way to tell when and if your exposure will lead to disease.

So-called "synergies" also are created in the environment and body that can exacerbate the effect of any single chemical. A synergy is simply a combination of two things that together, equal more than the sum of the individual parts. In straightforward mathematics, $1 + 1 = 2$ (no synergy here), but in the chemical world, $1 + 1$ can equal a lot more than 2 due to the interactive—synergistic—effect chemicals can have on one another. For example, on a scale of 1 to 10, Toxin A may be considered a 2 (low) while Toxin B is a 3, but together in the body they may cause a powerful, level 9 (high) effect. Synergies bring the number of potential chemical permutations to a nearly infinite amount. As Randall Fitzgerald notes in his book *The Hundred-Year Lie: How Food and Medicine Are Destroying Your Health* (2006), "What distresses and perplexes me is the realization that even if government had the resources to thoroughly conduct widespread safety testing—which it doesn't—our technology is too primitive to detect all of the synthetic chemicals in combination or to complete the task within our own lifetimes or even within the life spans of any of our grandchildren."

Fitzgerald goes on to share what Sheldon Krimsky calculated for his 2000 book, *Hormonal Chaos: The Scientific and Social Origins of the Environmental Endocrine Hypothesis*: If you take the most common one thousand chemicals and test them in unique combinations of three at a single dose per experiment, it would take 166 million different experiments to cover all the possibilities. And with up to 100,000 different synthetic chemicals in production and in the marketplace, the potential number of synergistic combinations becomes outrageous. Krimsky writes that it could take more than a thousand years to complete a full testing program, "an effort that would involve a level of complexity that could easily overwhelm our most advanced testing systems and surely our federal budget."

More than three thousand man-made chemicals get added to food products in the United States (for a variety of reasons: texture, taste, color, appearance, odor, flavor, or just to get you "addicted," as you'll see later on). Few of these chemicals have been tested in combination to investigate their potential synergistic effects in the body that can potentially be toxic to you.

When baker James Dewar invented the Twinkie in 1930, he used real ingredients—flour, sugar, salt, baking soda, eggs, and cream. Today's Twinkie has morphed into a scientific experiment; while Twinkies still do contain traces of the original ingredients, they also hold thirty-seven other ingredients that you won't find in your pantry. The creamy white filling is made mostly from partially hydrogenated vegetable oil and/or beef fat; polysorbate 60 is added to it, which is a gooey substance derived from corn, palm oil, and petroleum that helps replace cream and eggs at a fraction of the cost. Cellulose gum gives the filling a smooth, slippery feel. To get that vanilla flavor, they create it artificially in petrochemical plants. The cake part contains the emulsifier lecithin, a chemical that mimics the taste of butter (the real stuff would go rancid on a store shelf), and artificial dyes that give the cake the golden look of eggs. Sorbic acid, the only actual preservative in Twinkies, comes from petroleum.

THE INHALATIONS OF MODERN LIFE

The World Health Organization estimates that 4.6 million people die each year from causes directly attributable to air pollution, both indoor and outdoor. Worldwide more deaths per year are linked to air pollution than to automobile accidents. Health effects range from subtle biochemical and physiological changes to difficulty breathing; aggravation of existing respiratory and cardiac conditions; birth defects; damage to the immune, neurological, or reproductive system; and cancer.

In 2007, UCLA researchers published a stunning report that said exposure to a combination of diesel exhaust and high blood cholesterol increases the risk for heart attack and stroke far more than exposure to either factor alone. This is a perfect example of how toxins can have a deadly, synergistic effect—even with tissues or cells that are *not* themselves toxins. Adding diesel particles (1) to cholesterol fats (1) equals 3, not 2.

Cholesterol by itself is not a toxin, but this combination creates a dangerous interaction that wreaks cardiovascular havoc far beyond what is caused by either the diesel or cholesterol separately. It is now known that cholesterol is a marker of underlying inflammation.

Roughly 120 million Americans live in areas where the outdoor air is unhealthy. Air pollution comes from many different sources, such as factories, power plants, dry cleaners, cars, buses, trucks, and even windblown dust and wildfires. It can threaten the health of human beings, trees, lakes, crops, and animals, as well as damage the ozone layer and buildings. It also can cause haze, reducing visibility in national parks and wilderness areas. The substances that make up air pollution include gases such as sulfur dioxides, nitrogen oxides, hydrocarbons, and carbon monoxide; particulate matter such as smoke, dust, fumes, and aerosols; pesticides, chemicals, toxic elements, radioactive materials, and several other substances. These are considered primary air pollutants, meaning they are generated directly from a source or process. Then there are also secondary air pollutants formed in the air when primary pollutants react or interact. Ground-level ozone, which makes up photochemical smog, is a classic example of this. Some pollutants can be both primary and secondary; that is, they are both emitted directly and formed from other primary pollutants.

Of the 188 known air toxins, the top 33 that the EPA considers the greatest threat to human health are ever-present.

The 33 Most Hazardous Air Toxins

acetaldehyde	diesel particulate matter	nickel compounds
acrolein		perchloroethylene
acrylonitrile	ethylene dibromide	polychlorinated biphenyls (PCBs)
arsenic compounds	ethylene dichloride	
benzene	ethylene oxide	polycyclic organic matter (POM)
beryllium compounds	formaldehyde	
1, 3-butadiene	hexachlorobenzene	propylene dichloride
cadmium compounds	hydrazine	quinoline
carbon tetrachloride	lead compounds	1, 1, 2, 2-tetrachloroethane
chloroform	manganese compounds	
chromium compounds		trichloroethylene
coke oven emissions	mercury compounds	vinyl chloride
1, 3-dichloropropene	methylene chloride	

Source: Environmental Protection Agency

Classic Car Fumes

Let's take a pollutant that is getting more and more difficult to avoid: diesel particulate matter. Particulates are tiny particles of solid or liquid suspended in a gas, which is partly what comprises diesel exhaust. In addition, these soot particles also carry carcinogenic components such as benzopyrenes, aerosols such as ash particulates, metallic abrasion particles, sulfates, and silicates. All of these bode badly for the body. Exposure to diesel exhaust and its particulates is a known occupational hazard to truckers, railroad workers, and anyone using diesel-powered equipment. If we don't lighten up our commutes or take diesel-powered engines off the road, everyone can consider this a hazard.

How many of us have sat behind a truck or school bus and tried to hold our breath as we roll through the black cloud it leaves behind? There is perhaps no more common experience in America than the daily drives we take, whether it's to and from work or shuffling kids around. Today our daily commutes are breaking records. We average 25 minutes on the road per trip and millions of us (at last count, there were 3.4 million in 2000) are "extreme commuters"—traveling at least 90 minutes each way to get to work. And certainly there are millions more who are somewhere in between, especially people who live in suburbs of sprawling metropolises like Houston, Philadelphia, Los Angeles, New York, and Chicago. That's a lot of time driving in dirty air.

Nowadays we are more likely to drive cars that don't require diesel gas, but diesel-burning engines are still around us filling the air we breathe, from trucks and buses to roadside machinery and equipment that run on diesel gas (not to mention nearby factories and power plants). "Clean air" initiatives hope to reduce the number of diesel-burning engines on the road in the future, but we may still feel their effects for years to come—after they have been taken off the road. Because diesel particulates are so small, they can easily penetrate deep into the lungs once inhaled. The rough surfaces of these particles makes it easy for them to bind with other toxins in the environment, thus increasing the hazards of particle inhalation.

The EPA estimates that a proposed set of changes in diesel engine technology could result in 12,000 *fewer* premature mortalities, 15,000 *fewer* heart attacks, 6,000 *fewer* emergency room visits by children with asthma, and 8,900 *fewer* respiratory-related hospital admissions each year in the United States.

Not surprisingly, Los Angeles topped the American Lung Association's bad air 2007 list of most polluted cities in America. But there are signs of improvement: the number of days residents breathed the nation's worst ozone levels was fewer than in previous years. According to the EPA, the levels of six pollutants, including ozone and particulate matter, have declined 54 percent since 1970 in the city, when the Clean Air Act became law. Even as the national level of ozone, a key component of smog, declined, 99 million people in the United States still lived in counties with failing grades for ozone.

The Thrill of a New Car

Now that you have closed your car windows, let me ask you, have you ever wondered what makes a new car smell so *new*? Most of us have experienced the euphoria that comes with buying and getting into a brand new car fresh off the assembly line. The air inside new cars may contain some of the highest levels of vinyl chloride, which is used in the manufacture of automobile interiors. At room temperature, vinyl chloride releases dioxins in the air to produce that characteristic "new car" smell. Vinyl chloride, which is thought to be the most troubling kind of plastic from a health perspective, is also found in the discharge of exhaust gases from factories that manufacture or process vinyl chloride, or evaporation from areas where chemical wastes are stored. Most of the vinyl chloride produced in the United States is used to make polyvinyl chloride, or what we know as PVC.

Acute exposure in humans to vinyl chloride via inhalation has resulted in effects on the central nervous system, such as dizziness, drowsiness, headaches, and, yes, that "giddy" feeling, which is more or less a "high." Long-term effects can include liver damage and a set of symptoms that is actually termed "vinyl chloride disease," which includes joint and muscle pain, changes in the bones of your fingers, and thickening of the skin. Those sound like pretty common symptoms of people diagnosed with arthritis and scleroderma!

This points to the fact that it's not just outdoor air quality we need to worry about. Indoor air quality can be just as harmful, if not more so. In fact, the average indoor environment is actually *more* polluted, as it contains hazardous chemicals in concentrations 10 to 40 times greater than those outside. Indoor pollution typically comes from formaldehyde, aerosol spray products, air fresheners, asbestos, microbes and mold spores, carbon dioxide, house dust, cooking gas, colognes, and cleaning products. In a poorly ventilated building, these pollutants are concentrated and can give rise to a number of symptoms. Airborne chemicals can also come from lead-based paints, indoor pesticides (e.g., roach and ant killers), building materials and furnishings, chemically treated carpets, cabinetry or furniture made of certain pressed wood products, central heating and cooling systems, plasticizers, and tobacco smoke.

Asthma afflicts about 20 million Americans, including 6.3 million children. In 2000 there were nearly 2 million emergency room visits and nearly half a million hospitalizations due to asthma, at a cost of almost $2 billion, and causing 14 million missed school days each year. Studies confirm that indoor environmental factors contribute to the incidence of asthma. According to a World Health Report in 2002, indoor air pollution is responsible for 2.7 percent of the global burden of disease.

Formaldehyde's Hiding Places

We saw earlier how beds now contain a wide range of synthetics that give off gases for our bodies to absorb throughout the night. One of these gases is formaldehyde, which makes the EPA's top 33 list of most hazardous air toxins. It's used as a flame retardant in your mattress along with brominated substances that essentially build up in your body over time. Formaldehyde gas can cause several health problems, such as headaches, dizziness, nasal congestion, sore throat, scratchy eyes, coughing, and immune system abnormalities. Most fabrics treated with this flame retardant continuously emit this toxic gas, to the tune of 500 parts per million at the fabric's surface. And breathing just 0.1 parts per million for an extended time period can have health consequences. This is something to think about given that children's sleepwear is required by federal law to meet flammability standards.

Formaldehyde isn't confined to just your mattress. It's found in several household products, including disinfectants, bleach, aerosols, air fresheners, window and carpet cleaners, dry-cleaning fluids, and pesticides. The most significant source of formaldehyde in the indoor environment is probably pressed-wood products (particleboard, plywood, and fiberboard). It's been argued that the increase in childhood asthma in industrialized nations—tripling in just the last 30 years—could be attributed to the rise in formaldehyde's presence. What's more, children whose mothers use products in the home made of chemicals and that emit formaldehyde are more likely to develop asthma after birth. Once again, proof that babies in the womb are not as protected as we previously thought.

Many textile products have formaldehyde finishes. These include nylon and all polyester blends with permanent press fabrics. Synthetic carpets also contain formaldehyde, along with more than a dozen other hazardous chemicals (including xylene, benzene, and toluene), chemicals that continue to outgas from the carpets for up to five years after installation. The most dangerous stage of off-gassing is from four weeks to three months following installation. While carpets over five years old usually have stopped off-gassing, they may then become breeding grounds for dust mites and mold. Mold is a biological contaminant, rather than a chemical one, but it can give rise to damaging fungal toxins.

THE WASTE IN WATER

Water is essential to life, the life of the planet's ecosystems as well as to the human body. The pollution and toxicity of our oceans, lakes, waterways, ground water, and drinking water is having a devastating impact on our health and the health of our planet and wildlife. And you don't have to live near a beach that has closed down due to a toxic spill to be aware of the dangers or experience the effects of contaminated water.

Water supplies must originate from somewhere, but those sources are becoming infected with pollutants from a variety of places—power plants, factories, septic systems, sewage spills, waste disposal sites for hazardous materials that sink into the groundwater, animal feed lots, landfills, acid water runoff from mines, disposal wells, land disposal of sludge, spray irrigation, buried storage tanks and pipelines, and even from us dumping things down the drain like cosmetics and unused drugs. This list goes on and on. All these water contaminants in turn affect the food we eat because they become part of the soil and water supplies that ultimately nourish and grow our food.

Aquatic wildlife has taken a beating in the last several decades, and advances in technology are now giving us an unprecedented look at chemical contaminants in bodies of water throughout the United States and abroad. Among the most disturbing evidence of water pollution are the reports of sexually deformed and chemically castrated fish and amphibians. In several lakes and waterways, including the Great Lakes, Chesapeake Bay, the Columbia River in Washington, and the Potomac, fish have mutated into hermaphrodites (having both male and female sex organs) or changed sex entirely (gone from males to females). In southern California, many bottom-dwelling fish off the coast are now hermaphrodites. What's more, the ocean floor's sediment is contaminated with estrogenic chemicals that get absorbed by bottom-feeding organisms and passed up along the food chain. Chemicals that mimic the female hormone estrogen come from herbicides, fungicides, and pesticides that find their way to bodies of water. These then get incorporated into the biosystem that eventually becomes our water and food supplies. If these chemicals cause serious reproductive abnormalities and potential extinction in wildlife, what do they do to us?

In 2002, the first nationwide study of man-made chemicals and hormones in 139 streams revealed that 80 percent of streams tested were contaminated. Several of the chemicals examined are known or suspected of disrupting the hormone systems of animals and people. Of these, only a small fraction have been regulated at all, much less tested for toxicity, persistence in the environment, or other harmful characteristics, such as hormone disruption. Some of the same unregulated, widely used, hormone-disrupting chemicals have been detected at trace levels in the San Francisco Bay. In 2005, the United States Geological Survey found that by-products of common chemical products used by humans, including antibacterial soap, steroids, bug sprays, and prescription drugs, were entering streams and groundwater, causing a disruption to fish reproduction while increasing people's resistance to antibiotics when they consumed the fish.

As you can imagine, damage to the reproductive health of vulnerable fish populations may result in detrimental consequences to local fisheries and aquatic ecosystems; in addition, there is concern that people could become further exposed to hormone-disrupting chemicals by eating contaminated fish. So it's not just mercury that we need to concern ourselves with when it comes to seafood.

It's important to understand that hormones aren't just about those related to sex like estrogen and progesterone. A vast array of hormones control much of our bodily systems—from conception to death. They essentially set our metabolic processes in motion, and have as much to say about our reproductive system (and menstrual cycle for women) as they do about our hunger, ability to gain and lose weight, maintain a healthy immune system, keep a beating heart, recover from injury, think clearly, sleep soundly, have a general sense of well-being, and so much more. If you disrupt your body's natural hormonal state, you throw your entire body out of whack and leave it vulnerable to an onslaught of health problems, from minor to life-threatening.

When Drinking Water Is Dangerous

A minimal amount of drinking water contamination is to be expected as a result of natural processes; however, today's tap water, whether coming from municipal water supplies or private wells, from surface water or underground aquifers, is much more than minimally contaminated.

Contaminants in drinking water may be either chemical or microbial. Microbial contaminants, such as viruses, bacteria, and parasites, come from human and animal waste. An outbreak of the microscopic parasite *Cryptosporidium* in the Milwaukee water supply in 1993 killed 400 people and sickened some 400,000. But chemicals are the most likely hazard, and more than 700 chemicals have been identified in American drinking water. These include asbestos, pesticides, heavy metals, industrial waste, nitrates, and a variety of chemicals, including by-products created from the use of disinfecting agents and those known to be carcinogenic. The EPA only monitors 84 out of the 2,100 contaminants found in drinking water, and a significant number of violations of the standards set for these 84 contaminants have been reported since the Safe Drinking Water Act was first enacted in 1974.

One of the most surprising discoveries of late has been the detection of perchlorate in 160 public water systems in 22 states, which urged the Environmental Working Group to publish a press release in 2006 declaring perchlorate a "widespread public health threat" for pregnant women. The vast majority of perchlorate manufactured in the United States is used by the Department of Defense to make solid rocket and missile fuel, while smaller amounts are used to make fireworks and road flares. Perchlorate is also a contaminant of certain types of fertilizer that were widely used in the early part of the twentieth century but are in limited use today. In addition to water supplies, perchlorate has also been found in a wide variety of domestic and imported produce. Tests by the CDC and independent researchers have confirmed that virtually all Americans carry some level of perchlorate in their bodies, and that many have levels well above the levels found to lower thyroid levels.

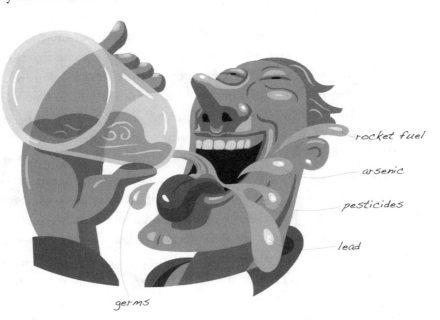

rocket fuel

arsenic

pesticides

lead

germs

What's in Your Water? Pollution, old pipes, and outdated treatment can render tap water harmful, even though you can't see, taste, or smell the contaminants. Up to 7 million Americans become sick from dirty tap water each year. Bottled water fares no better; about one-fourth of bottled water is bottled tap water (and by some accounts, as much as 40 percent is derived from tap water). Popular brands of bottled water have tested positive for elevated levels of arsenic, bacteria, and other impurities. According to the Natural Resources Defense Council (www.nrdc.org), one brand of "spring water" whose label pictured a lake and mountains, actually came from a well in an industrial facility's parking lot, near a hazardous waste dump. It was periodically contaminated with industrial chemicals at levels above FDA standards (mind you, the bottled water industry is largely unregulated in the United States). Simple solution: filter your tap water.

Bottled water companies have made a killing in the last decade as people turn to them for convenience, purity, or even fashion. The surprise: most bottled water is still just tap water, but unlike tap water, bottled water is not regulated. And, to make matters worse, the plastic bottles it comes in often leach chemicals into the water. The bottles are often made of PVC (polyvinyl chloride), an environmental hazard itself. A four-year study conducted by the nonprofit Natural Resources Defense Council found contaminants in one-third of bottled water samples to exceed EPA tap water standards. Other independent studies have discovered fluoride, phthalates, trihalomethanes, and arsenic in bottled water, coming either from the bottling process or from the bottles themselves. Environmental groups are also concerned about the amount of waste that these plastic bottles create.

While one might assume that really bad water would be self-evident by way of its smell or taste, sadly the most devastating stories of unexplained illness and disease in pockets of communities across the country often don't become front-page material until enough bodies have been collected and curiosity has mounted. In 2000 the hit movie *Erin Brockovich* was based on one woman's crusade to prove that a chemical leak into the groundwater of a small town led to a disturbing array of health problems in the community. Another case that made headlines recently involved a military base at Camp Lejeune in North Carolina, where 75,000 Marines and their families were exposed to toxic tap water that may have caused cancer and birth defects. Federal hearings took place in the summer of 2007, and numerous residents of the base testified about their personal horror stories—children born with severe disabilities or disorders, and many who later died of unusual cancers.

Are Chlorine and Fluoride a Problem?

Two of the most damaging substances, both to overall health and to digestive function, found abundantly in the water supply are chlorine and fluoride. This identification of fluoride as a pollutant may come as a shock to some, for we have been led to believe that it is an essential nutrient needed to prevent tooth decay, not a water pollutant. The fact of the matter is that the EPA has set a Maximum Contaminant Level (an enforceable standard set for drinking water contaminants) for fluoride, substantiating that it is, indeed, a contaminant. To make matters worse, the form of fluoride used in water fluoridation programs is an industrial waste product. More than 90 percent of the fluoridated U.S. municipal water supplies use hydrofluorosilicic acid or its sodium salt as a fluoridating agent. These chemicals are highly toxic by-products of phosphate fertilizer production. Their presence in our drinking water supplies is more about the corporate bottom line than about the claimed benefit of preventing tooth decay. The appalling aspect of this whole scenario is the adverse health affects that can result from fluoride exposure, even at the relatively low doses used in water fluoridation programs. These may include

- **hyperactivity**
- **learning disabilities**
- **cancer**
- **hypothyroidism**
- **dental fluorosis (permanent discoloration of teeth) in children**
- **arthritis**
- **kidney disease**
- **gastrointestinal disorders**
- **birth defects**
- **lowered immunity**

Links to studies verifying the role of fluoride in these disorders and others may be found at http://www.slweb.org/bibliography.html, a Web site founded by Fluoride Action Network, a group formed in 2000 by scientists (including EPA scientists), dentists, and environmentalists to educate the public on the toxicity of fluoride compounds and the health impacts of current fluoride exposures.

Chlorine, added as a disinfectant to water, becomes a problem when it unites with other pollutants and/or organic matter, such as decaying vegetation, to form trihalomethanes (ThMs). These compounds include such deadly chemicals as chloroform, bromoform, and carbon tetrachloride, all of which have been linked with increased incidences of atherosclerosis, colon and rectal cancer, and bladder cancer. Chlorinated water also destroys much of our beneficial intestinal flora, needed to protect us from pathogens.

Drugged Drinking Water

Pharmaceutical drugs prescribed at high rates such as antidepressants and antibiotics are now turning up in rivers and groundwater. In addition to people dumping excess or expired prescription drugs down the drain or toilet, pharmaceuticals are also making their way into drinking water through human waste *after* people take these drugs. They enter sewage treatment centers, which don't weed out these chemicals before drinking water is processed. This phenomenon is not limited to the United States; England got its first dose of this reality a few years ago when scientists looked at 12 pharmaceuticals thought to pose an environmental threat, including painkillers, antibiotics, and antidepressants, and found traces of these pharmaceuticals in both sewage waters and drinking water. They also found traces in the rivers downstream from sewage treatment plants. No doubt this could be one of the reasons why ocean life is continuing to decline around the world, and it seems as if it won't be very long at all before these prescription drug pollutants start showing up in shellfish such as shrimp, crab, and lobsters, and maybe even in seaweed someday.

Pharmaceutical chemicals are not regulated by the Environmental Protection Agency, so there is no enforced limit of pharmaceuticals in the drinking water. In fact, in the United States, there is no government agency that is even testing the level of pharmaceuticals in public drinking water on a regular basis. So it is possible, in fact likely, that these levels will continue to rise in the years ahead without being detected or reported to the public at all. I often think about the environmental impact of our culture's massive consumption levels of prescription drugs. Currently this is an underacknowledged area of study that will surely take on a more prominent place in research and public health circles. I don't want to imagine a day when the fish market is selling "Prozac-free perch."

FORMULAIC FOOD

If there's one thing humans have perfected in the last century, it's how to process food and create flavors and additives exclusively from chemicals that make many common foods taste the way they do. In fact, food production outpaced population growth over the last forty years, and about 90 percent of the money that Americans spend on food is used to buy processed food. Whether you live in a sprawling metropolis or a small town in the middle of America, you probably don't have to go too far to find a fast food restaurant, or at least a convenience store that sells mostly processed foods. We also have entered an era of genetically modified foods, which are just that—genetically *mutated* foods that are not necessarily better for you. The health implications not only to humans but also to the environment is a hotly contested debate; the introduction of genetically altered food could have serious consequences, such as allergic reactions and increased resistance to certain antibiotics. Two of the prime targets for genetic engineering—soy and corn—are America's cash crops. These are among the accomplices in our largely overprocessed food supply, entering our diets as ingredients in processed foods.

The infiltration of fast food into our lives—and its economic, cultural, and health consequences—was expertly described in chilling detail in Eric Schlosser's best-selling book *Fast Food Nation: The Dark Side of the All-American Meal*. Schlosser gives an incisive history of the development of American fast food, drawing alarming conclusions about how we have come to face epidemic obesity and toxic, sometimes lethal, food sources, and generally how the fast food industry has changed the landscape of how Americans eat and live. On any given day, one out of four Americans opts for a quick and inexpensive meal at a fast food restaurant, without giving either its speed or its thriftiness a second thought. According to *Time* magazine, 70 percent of kids ages six to eight think fast food is healthier than home food. Fast food spending by consumers has increased eighteen-fold since 1970. A typical hamburger in 1957 weighed 1 ounce and contained 210 calories. Today, that same hamburger is 6 ounces and packs 618 calories. What's worse: 25 percent of the vegetables eaten in the United States are french fries.

Despite the choices you have every day over what you eat and what you do, the mere convenience and reliability of fast food—and even processed foods found at local markets—has programmed many Americans in a way that makes eating this food a mindless act. That is, people eat these foods without thinking about what they are doing or how it will affect them in the long run. The last time you ordered from a fast food giant or bought a grab-and-go lunchbox from a corner store, did you think about where the food came from or how it was made? Probably not. You unwrapped your food and dug right in.

Among the chilling details uncovered by Schlosser are the current methods for preparing fast food (and, for that matter, processed foods in general), which are less likely to be found in cookbooks than in trade journals such as *Food Technologist* and *Food Engineering*. The scientists behind the development of the industry for fast and processed food, which took off after World War II, knew less about nutrition than they did about making products taste better, last longer, and be safe from contamination by microorganisms. The industry made calories affordable and available, at the expense of our health. And at the expense of natural food's nutritive components. All that technology behind taste, shelf life, and (ironically) "safety" means processing and altering natural foods to the point that they contain few nutrients, and many preservatives, chemicals, sodium, and so on. Think about the evolution of the Twinkie.

The Artifice in "Artificial" and "Natural" Flavor

There's not much of a difference between "artificial flavoring" and "natural flavors" in processed food. Both are man-made additives that give processed food most of its taste. A natural flavor isn't necessarily healthier or purer than an artificial one. Natural and artificial flavors are manufactured at the same chemical plants, and sometimes they contain the exact same chemicals, produced through different methods. For example, amyl acetate gives the dominant note of banana flavor. When you distill it from bananas with a solvent, amyl acetate is a natural flavor. But when you produce it by mixing vinegar with amyl alcohol, and using sulfuric acid as a catalyst, you get amyl acetate as an artificial flavor.

Not surprisingly, the flavor industry is highly secretive. Legend has it that a German scientist discovered methyl anthranilate, one of the first artificial flavors, by accident while mixing chemicals in the laboratory. The lab suddenly filled with the sweet smell of grapes, and voilà! Methyl anthranilate soon became the main ingredient in grape Kool-Aid.

Flavor companies are huge plants comprised of a small and elite group of skilled scientists ("food technologists" or "flavorists") who work in labs to find the right chemical balance in test tubes to give you the flavor of those french fries, and even the flavor in toothpastes, ice cream, breakfast cereals, chips, pet food, cookies, mouthwashes, antacids, soft drinks, sports drinks, bottled teas, wine coolers, all-natural juice drinks, organic soy drinks, beers, and malt liquors. These same plants manufacture the smells found in fine perfumes, as well as household products (e.g., deodorant, dishwashing detergent, bath soap, shampoo, furniture polish, floor wax). The process is the same: food and aroma technologists manipulate volatile chemicals to create particular tastes and smells. So, as Schlosser puts it, "The basic science behind the scent of your shaving cream is the same as that governing the flavor of your TV dinner."

> **FACT**
>
> The American flavor industry has annual revenues of about $1.4 billion. Approximately 10,000 new processed food products are introduced every year in the United States. Almost all of them require flavor additives.

Colorful Science

Giving food the right color is also a science. Color additives make food more appealing. They are more prevalent in common foods than you think, too. At the major fast food chains, color additives are added to soft drinks, salad dressings, cookies, condiments, chicken dishes, and sandwich buns. But the fast food industry isn't solely to blame, as food additives are found in just about everything these days. Many strawberry yogurts, for example, get their color from carmine, which is also found in many frozen fruit bars, candies, fruit fillings, and juice drinks, as well as cosmetics like lipstick and eye shadow. Carmine is a food dye derived from ground-up insects that produce the pigment-containing carminic acid. (As with many food additives, carmine is not required by the FDA to be explicitly named in all ingredient lists, and may sometimes be represented under "natural coloring" or "added coloring." It has been known to cause severe allergic reactions and anaphylactic shock in some people.)

The notion that food could have an effect on children's behavior became popularized in the 1970s by allergist Benjamin Feingold, M.D., who published the Feingold diet. To treat hyperactivity, he advocated a diet free of more than three hundred food additives. While his ideas have been challenged ever since, studies continue to emerge that bolster the argument and point to the damaging effects food additives can have when consumed heavily. In addition to attention problems, synthetic food additives have been linked to restlessness, irritability, aggressiveness, and excitability in young children. There is something to be said for the joke about "drinking the Kool-Aid"—most fruit drinks owe their flavor (and popularity) to chemicals that can trigger disruptive behaviors. Infants are particularly sensitive to chemical food colorings, flavorings, and preservatives because their organs may not be fully developed at birth. And fetuses whose mothers are consuming food with additives are perhaps the worst off; they can face health problems years later and into adulthood that are rooted in cellular changes brought on by exposure to those chemicals during that vulnerable life stage.

Sufficiently Sugared

Nutritional deficiencies result whenever tissues are deprived of adequate amounts of essential nutrients over a period of time. Researchers have examined blood samples, for example, of children diagnosed with attention or learning problems, looking for deficiencies in vitamins, minerals, or other nutrients. The theory: distracted children don't absorb nutrients properly or get sufficient nutrients in their diets. Some studies have found low levels of healthy fats required by the body; other studies have discovered deficiencies in minerals, such as iron or zinc. Children who take supplements to make up for a specific shortfall become noticeably more settled in school or at home.

In 2004 researchers told a United Nations panel that dietary shortages of crucial vitamins and minerals like zinc and iron may be keeping as many as a third of the world's people from reaching their full potential; as many as one-fifth of the world's population lack enough zinc in their diets, putting children in particular at risk of dwarfism, diarrhea, and serious respiratory infections such as pneumonia.

Symptoms of a nutritional deficiency are not necessarily obvious. Associated conditions develop slowly over time and can be very insidious and difficult to identify. You don't need to have scurvy to have a vitamin C deficiency. (Here's an eye-opener: in the last twenty-five years the level of vitamin C deficiency in our population has gone from 3 to 5 percent to a confounding 20 percent—largely due to the shift from whole foods to processed foods.) Vitamin C is essential to your body's breakdown and utilization of food, and the body can neither manufacture it on its own or store it. By the same token, you don't need to have osteoporosis to have a

It's amazing what you can do without any help from drugs.

calcium deficiency, yet millions don't get enough calcium on a daily basis as a result of diet choices. Symptoms can be as subtle as appetite loss, bad breath, soft or brittle fingernails, fatigue, insomnia, general weakness, inability to recover from injury or illness quickly, impotence, and easy bruising.

The reason I point out the trend in nutrient and vitamin deficiency is because it relates directly to the body's ability to ward off illness, disease, and operate completely to combat incoming toxins. When you don't equip your body with the tools it needs to support its internal structures and functions, it won't be able to withstand the environment in which you live. And it could rebel in unexpected ways as your body burden gets bigger, and literally heavier.

When a doctor sees a "fatty liver" or, worse, the beginnings of cirrhosis, in a patient, he is likely to start asking questions about alcohol consumption. (A person who has fat in the liver but no inflammation or liver damage is said to have a "fatty liver"; this condition can progress to cirrhosis, which is characterized by a liver that is permanently damaged, scarred, and no longer able to work properly.)

But more and more doctors are now getting an unexpected response:

"Doc, I don't drink alcohol. I don't even smoke." And some of these patients are children—about one in ten kids are showing signs of being an alcoholic. But clearly they aren't drinkers. After careful examination, the doctor has a diagnosis: nonalcoholic steatohepatitis or NASH. This is a common, often "silent" liver disease that resembles alcoholic liver disease, but occurs in people who drink little or no alcohol. The major feature in NASH is fat in the liver, along with inflammation and damage. Most people with NASH feel well and are not aware that they have a liver problem. Nevertheless, NASH can be severe and can lead to cirrhosis. The guilty party? Too much processed food and sugar.

> **FACT**
>
> NASH affects 2 to 5 percent of Americans. An additional 10 to 20 percent of Americans have fat in their liver, but no inflammation or liver damage, a condition called "fatty liver." NASH ranks as one of the major causes of cirrhosis in America, behind hepatitis C and alcoholic liver disease.

Scientists are beginning to see more cases of NASH as obesity numbers climb; in the past ten years, the rate of obesity has doubled in adults and tripled in children. This has also led some doctors to point fingers at refined sugar as if it were as bad as alcohol in its destructive behavior on the liver (not to mention other body parts and systems). The progression of NASH can take years, even decades. The process can stop and, in some cases, reverse on its own without specific therapy (but likely with some diet and lifestyle changes). Or NASH can slowly worsen, causing scarring or "fibrosis" to appear and accumulate in the liver. As fibrosis worsens, cirrhosis develops; the liver becomes seriously scarred, hardened, and unable to function normally. Not every person with NASH develops cirrhosis, but once serious scarring or cirrhosis is present, few treatments can halt the progression.

Among the suspected causes of NASH are insulin resistance, the release of toxic inflammatory proteins by fat cells (cytokines), and oxidative stress (deterioration of cells) inside liver cells. All of these underlying causes can be linked back to lifestyle choices that exacerbate these conditions. People with NASH are recommended to reduce their weight if obese or overweight, follow a balanced and healthy diet, increase physical activity, and avoid toxins that strain the liver. All of these steps are basic features of the RENEW program. It's amazing what you can do without any help from drugs or pharmaceuticals to turn a condition like NASH—or diabetes, for that matter—around. The principles of RENEW will help you get on that path of wellness.

THE PERILS OF CONVENIENCE

How many of us readily buy canned goods, use nonstick coated pots and pans, and have untold ways of using plastic in the kitchen—from soft sandwich bags to hard storage containers and bottles? We owe a lot of these conveniences of modern life to advancements in chemical configurations and designs. But at a potential hidden human cost: bisphenol A (BPA), a plastic and resin ingredient used to make a wide variety of plastic goods and to line metal food and drink cans (ever wonder how those canned contents slip so easily out and onto your plate, or into your bowl or mouth?), is a toxin associated with birth defects of the male and female reproductive systems. BPA is commonplace—found in copious brands of fruit, vegetables, soda, and other frequently eaten canned goods. It migrates from the can or plastic into the contents, which are then ingested.

What's most troubling about the recent reports of BPA's prevalence, which emerged in 2007 and was featured prominently in the media, is that it remains entirely without safety standards. It is allowed in unlimited amounts in consumer products, drinking water, and food, the top exposure source for most people. The lack of enforceable limits has resulted in widespread contamination of canned foods at levels that pose potential risks.

Modern-day pots and pans fare no better in their chemical makeup. When you use a Teflon-coated pan or storage unit (perhaps to avoid the legendary toxin aluminum underneath), you could be trading convenience for toxicity. Unfortunately, Teflon is one of the hardiest man-made products, its molecules surviving forever in the environment and in your body. When heated, Teflon's chemical off-gassing will kill some birds if they are in the same room.

Aluminum has had a long history, from fables that it can cause Alzheimer's to facts that it's a powerful neurotoxin damaging to brain cells. Yet it can be found in numerous products, including vaccines routinely given to children. Almost all food and water supplies contain some amount of aluminum, for

FACT

BPA is at unsafe levels in one of every ten servings of canned foods (11 percent) and one of every three cans of infant formula (33 percent). BPA, found in everything from baby bottles and water cooler jugs to bicycle helmets, CDs, and the inside lining of tin cans, is associated with a number of health problems and diseases that are on the rise in the United States population, including breast and prostate cancers and infertility.

it is used by municipal water supplies as a "flocculating" agent to remove dirt, and it is widely used in food processing. In addition to cookware, it is also found in foil and utensils, antiperspirants, paints, cosmetics, and baking powders, as well as over-the-counter painkillers, anti-inflammatory drugs, antacids, and douche preparations.

CAUGHT OFF GUARD

Last year, we saw an unprecedented number of recalls happen in the toy market. As I write this, Mattel, the world's largest toy company, is trying to scrub its tarnished image clean after several high-profile recalls on toys manufactured in China that may contain poisonous levels of lead in their paint. By the beginning of September 2007 close to a dozen popular toys around the world, including eight playsets sold under the Barbie brand and three Fisher-Price toys, were pulled from the shelves. In a little more than a month, Mattel recalled more than 21 million of these toys worldwide. Disney then announced it would start conducting independent testing on its toys that feature Disney characters.

While the recalls help avert the consequences of exposing millions of children and their families to potentially dangerous levels of lead (and possibly other toxins), what's disconcerting about these recalls is how they expose a "hidden harm." You cannot necessarily see, taste, feel, or sense a toxic level of lead in an otherwise harmless child's toy. We assume a company as established and esteemed as Mattel would have a superior method for testing products for safety (and, by the same token, that the Consumer Product Safety Commission would be an added shield). What these recalls do is diminish our confidence in consumer products and the people who are supposed to protect us from injurious goods ever reaching our local stores. Congress is now investigating the recalls, but again, this only goes to show another example of treating a problem rather than preventing it. It's stepping in after the fact. How much irreversible harm has already been done?

The Mattel cases caught many unsuspecting parents off guard. Amid the toy recalls came another report that said some garden hoses may contain dangerous levels of lead. In one particular test, some Phoenix reporters purchased ten garden hoses at familiar home improvement and hardware stores. After filling sections of the hoses with clean water, sealing the ends, and putting them outside for about a day, they then brought that water to a lab. What they discovered was astonishing: five of the ten hoses came back with levels of lead higher than what the EPA allows for drinking water, which is 15 parts per billion.

Between the Mattel recalls and coverage by *ABC News* of the garden hose story, the cry for a stronger national standard on lead in all products is growing louder. We should not be caught off guard with reports after the fact, especially when it comes to the safety of children in their critical developmental years. After all, there is only so much we can do as consumers once products land in our pockets and homes. Hopefully the latest waves of recalls and "unexpected" findings heighten the global concern about the safety of *all* products no matter where they are made.

Chapter 9 Summary

- By looking at the common ingredients of modern life—from plush mattresses, stain-resistant carpets, and wrinkle-free clothing to personal care products, cars, and crowded highways—we see how we can come into contact with more toxins than we ever thought possible. The average adult uses about nine personal care products a day, totaling about 126 chemicals. At least one-third of these ingredients have been noted to cause cancer or some other serious health problem.

- Three common myths we falsely believe are 1) that the government would not let us be exposed to anything harmful; 2) that labels tell the whole story; and 3) that toxins are harmless in small amounts.

- Synergies are the interactions that occur when two or more toxins are combined. The synergy of two weak toxins can combine to have a dangerous effect that's much greater than the sum of those two single toxins.

- Hidden harms exist everywhere. Surprising sources of toxins include

  - pharmaceutical drugs and rocket fuel in drinking water
  - formaldehyde in household goods and furniture
  - untold additives in food
  - plastics and resins in commonly used bottles, cans, and storage containers that leach a noxious chemical
  - toys made with lead paint

- Too much sugar, especially from processed foods, can do as much damage to the liver as excess alcohol. About one in ten children today show signs of a fatty liver, which is also attributed to rising levels of obesity. This condition is reversible through diet and lifestyle changes.

CHAPTER 10

DETOXIFICATION AND YOUR HEALTH

❧

It's no surprise that detoxification has become a prominent treatment as people have become more aware of pollution, both in the general environment and from things like consumer products and common household cleaning agents. It is estimated that one in every four Americans suffers from some level of heavy metal poisoning. Heavy metals, such as lead, mercury, cadmium, and arsenic, are by-products of industry. Synthetic agriculture chemicals, many of which are known to cause health problems, are also found in food, air, and water. American agriculture uses nearly ten pounds (4.5 kg) of pesticides per person on the food supply each year. These toxins have become almost unavoidable. Pesticides that are used only on crops in the southern United States have been found in the tissue of animals in the far north of Canada. DDT, a cancer-causing insecticide that has been banned for decades, is still regularly found in the fatty tissue of animals, birds, and fish, even in extremely remote regions such as the North Pole.

❧

Toxins that are stored in the body can eventually overwhelm the liver. The result of this toxic overload is inflammation, which leads to chronic conditions such as heart disease, diabetes, obesity, cancer, Alzheimer's, Parkinsonism, and autoimmune diseases. In other words, chronic low-grade systemic inflammation is likely the foundation of most all diseases. Because toxins are foreign substances, the body will try to erect a barrier between them and its own cells, organs, and tissues. This barrier is inflammation, the body's attempt to protect itself from these toxic foreign substances. Inflammation can occur anywhere in the body where toxins are present. For example, if they are present in the joints, the result may be arthritis; if present in the colon, the result may be colitis. Even with diet improvements and a decrease in the impact of environmental toxins, the toxins that are stored in the body will remain there until removed. This is accomplished with detoxification and cleansing.

As you've been learning since the beginning of this book, toxins can be sneaky about how they get into your body, sit quietly for years, and eventually reveal themselves through sudden or chronic illness in the long term. At that point it may be too difficult to "turn back the clock" and reverse the effects that those toxins have had. It's like having a million dollars in your bank account after steadily nourishing your account for years; it took time for that money to grow and compound, and you can't just get back that time in an instant. The secret to having a healthy long life and increasing your longevity is in nourishing your body every day routinely year after year. Just as sudden windfalls of cash are not likely in the real world, so is a sudden gift of health without any effort or self-care on your part on a daily basis. I can't express how powerful just a few slight shifts in your lifestyle can be to help limit your exposure to toxins and get you on that path. And you will feel like a million bucks!

When you consider the extent to which we suffer from chronic and life-threatening diseases while living in one of the richest, most medically advanced countries in the world, you have to wonder where we are going wrong—and where we could be doing better. Sadly, with progress and technology come the consequence—toxic waste. And with an increase of environmental toxins comes an increase in the risk for health problems, notably those that gain momentum with continued exposure and worsen over time as the body begins to rebel in unexpected ways. Eventually, a nagging illness sets in.

The statistics continue to be staggering. Nearly 20 million Americans have diabetes, which is the sixth-leading cause of death in the United States (and largely preventable); millions more are prediabetic and don't even know it. Almost 50 million suffer from chronic diseases such as asthma or lupus; about 70 million have arthritis, the leading cause of disability in the United States. Childhood asthma has increased by more than 40 percent since 1980, making asthma one of the most prevalent illnesses affecting us as a society today. And though several factors may be at play for this increase, environmental scientists are now looking at the combination of prolonged exposure to artificial chemicals and a nutrient-deficient diet. At the heart of asthma is a troubled immune system that cannot tolerate certain substances. So many toxins can infiltrate and confuse our immune system that it's no wonder the rise in asthma has correlated with a rise in environmental toxins.

Fifteen years ago, a half million Americans had Alzheimer's disease. Today 5 million Americans have it, a number totally out of proportion to the population increase. This fact makes sense, given so many chemicals that are known to cause widespread brain-damage.

For me, the most eye-opening statistic is this: *All* of us carry toxins in our bodies that Mother Nature never intended us to bear. One hundred percent of us—no matter where or how we live—are laced with chemical pollutants that are suspected to cause cancer, disrupt hormone functioning, or lead to birth abnormalities. Most of these chemicals come directly from common consumer goods and food—not field trips to farms or accidents in a college chem lab. Whether we like it or not, we have to accept this fact and do what we can to address it. On a positive note, this will ultimately get us to where we want to be: a state of optimum physical, mental, and emotional health.

In this chapter I want to take more time to describe and detail some of the chemical connections between toxins and our bodies that will interest those who want more information. While I've explained many of the health problems that correlate with a toxic overload, now we turn to the spectrum of problems as they relate to individual *systems* in the body. I hope this chapter helps you further see how vital it is that you take charge of your body today and to help it continually renew itself on a daily basis. Having an understanding of each system as it relates to the whole unit that is the magical human body, you will come to appreciate the value in detoxification and cleansing. You will also gain new insights on taking care of that one body you have in order to live life to its fullest.

THE DIGESTIVE SYSTEM

The health of your digestive system may not be at the forefront of your mind each day, but it is undoubtedly something that none of us can afford to ignore. I know that amid the hectic pace of everyday living, an occasional bout of heartburn or constipation is often easy to overlook, but some gastrointestinal problems can lead to other, more serious, issues if not addressed. When it was discovered more than twenty years ago that my own battle with weight gain and poor health was the result of a poorly functioning digestive system, I knew I had to make a change. I promised myself that I would do whatever was necessary to regain control of my body and my health, and it was during that personal healing process that I discovered the natural remedies that would become the foundation for my recovery. Since then, I have made it my personal mission to educate others about the importance of proper digestion.

The effect toxins can have on the body's capacity to efficiently absorb nutrients, eliminate waste, and fuel the engines of human life is especially important to me as a digestive health expert. In my experience, digestive health is the center of gravity for all other points of health in the body. When out of balance, sick, or diseased, virtually every other system and organ gets negatively affected, triggering scores of problems you wouldn't normally or intuitively link directly to the digestive tract.

Irritable bowel syndrome (IBS) is one of the most common intestinal disorders, affecting about 10 to 15 percent of people in North America. Up to 20 percent of people have symptoms of IBS, such as abdominal pain and altered bowel habits, although less than half of them see a doctor for their symptoms. IBS is an elusive ailment, one I call a "trash basket diagnosis" because people who have GI complaints that don't match any specific diagnosis are often told they have the condition. Examples of symptoms include abdominal pain, diarrhea and constipation, gas, nausea, bloating, heartburn, excessive excretion of mucus from the colon, fatigue, some degree of anxiety or depression, and bowel urgency or incontinence. A more serious condition not necessarily resulting from IBS is inflammatory bowel *disease*, which causes ongoing inflammation of the intestines and includes ulcerative colitis and Crohn's disease. Inflammatory bowel disease affects fewer people and tends to be hereditary.

Notable with IBS is the fact that it is strictly a functional disorder, with no identified structural defects. Though IBS sufferers often seek medical help and rarely require hospitalization, the symptoms can significantly interfere with normal daily activities. If you are personally familiar with IBS, then you know very well how much it can put a damper on quality of life. There are many studies that conclude that the constant intake of food additives and the ingestion of pesticides, chemicals, and dyes can cause irritation to the intestinal tract and/or an imbalance of the intestinal microflora, resulting in inflammation or symptoms of irritable bowel syndrome.

When I utter the world *constipation* in a roomful of people, it's always interesting to watch the response. Constipation is not something we usually like to talk about in public. But it's a common complaint, and a very important topic, as proper bowel function is one of the main channels of toxin elimination. A sluggish colon means a sluggish liver, and vice versa. A liver that is not functioning to capacity and perhaps not producing enough bile may in fact contribute to constipation. Chronic constipation can also be a result of a constant intake of toxic elements as well as food choices that are processed and full of preservatives. A diet of processed foods can leave a person lacking essential nutrients needed by the liver for detoxification. Bad food choices can also leave you lacking a good amount of fiber. Fiber is needed to absorb the waste and toxins that the liver is sending to the intestines to hopefully get them out of the body. Chronic constipation can result in the reabsorption of bacteria, digestive toxins, and chemical wastes into the bloodstream, once again taxing the liver.

I mentioned earlier that a stressed-out liver may not be able to operate at full capacity and effectively process all the toxins and materials it encounters. We also have seen how excess toxin intake, to which we are all subjected, puts excess stress on the liver. It can also instigate an imbalance in the liver detox system itself that can lead to the storage of toxic materials. Remember: when phase I reactions are more active than phase II reactions, the accumulation of active intermediaries can lead to tissue damage and disease. Over a period of time, such a pattern can result in the development of chemical sensitivities, where people are oversensitive to environmental toxins. If either phase I or phase II—or both—become overloaded, toxins will accumulate in the body, especially in fatty tissue, where they may remain for life. The brain and endocrine (hormonal) glands are common sites for toxic accumulation, which can result in brain dysfunction and hormonal imbalances, giving rise to a number of cognitive, emotional, and physical problems.

This can contribute to inflammation of the liver, also called hepatitis. Yes, there are forms of hepatitis not caused by a virus. As we saw, there are forms of liver disease caused by a toxic overload of nutrient-poor foods. People who don't smoke or drink alcohol yet consume too much sugar and processed foods have been shown to develop fatty livers that can progress to cirrhosis. Hepatitis can also result from an autoimmune response, in which the immune system overreacts and begins to attack the liver's healthy cells. The immune system, of course, is fighting foreign invaders including both pathogens as well as chemicals. Cirrhosis of the liver can be a direct result of continued damage and inflammation as well as the intake of too much alcohol.

THE RESPIRATORY SYSTEM

Asthma's 20 million victims, including more than 6 million children, may want to scrutinize their breathing spaces closely. Plenty of research exists to support the relationship between air pollution and asthma and, for that matter, pollution and allergies, which affect *20 percent* of Americans (60 million people). Other than natural triggers like pollen and dust, pollutants that trigger asthma and allergies can be found in both indoor and outdoor environments—pesticides, tobacco, soot, car exhaust, engine fuel, cleaning supplies, and any man-made chemical used to manufacture consumer products or "protect" things such as furniture, upholstery, mattresses, and carpets.

It's no surprise that we've seen a corresponding rise in allergies with a rise in environmental toxins. This can set off a double whammy—compromising the immune system and activating it (or in some cases, *deactivating* it) to the point that you open yourself up to a host of health problems. Allergies are hallmarks of an immune system out of whack. The more toxins you load into the system, the more likely you can exacerbate your allergies and become more allergic to more things. Constant overexposure and the resulting constant immune reaction in the body is not a recipe for long-term health. But, with proper detoxification, you may be able to decrease (or perhaps eliminate) allergic reactions. This has the added benefit of boosting your immune system and allowing it to be strong when true pathogens like viruses and bacteria enter.

Chronic obstructive pulmonary disease (COPD) is an umbrella term for people with chronic bronchitis, emphysema, or both. In this condition, the airflow to the lungs is restricted (obstructed). COPD is usually a result of smoking, but air pollution, polluted work areas, or simply long-term exposure to certain airborne chemicals can be causative agents. This is what many of the workers at the 9/11 site in New York City are now dealing with. According to a study published in the *American Journal of Respiratory and Critical Care Medicine*, workers at the World Trade Center site had a decline in lung function a year later that was equivalent to twelve years of aging-related pulmonary decline.

THE CARDIOVASCULAR SYSTEM

Heart disease remains the number one killer of both men and women, affecting an estimated 62 million Americans—more than any other illness. It's common knowledge that lack of exercise and poor diet increase one's risk for developing heart disease or having a heart attack, but few people stop to consider other risks involved. Cardiovascular disease has been linked to air pollution, and toxicity from heavy metals such as lead and cadmium. According to the American Heart Association, "epidemiological studies conducted worldwide have shown a consistent, increased risk for cardiovascular events, including heart and stroke deaths, in relation to short- and long-term exposure to present-day concentrations of pollution, especially particulate matter."

A 2007 edition of the online journal *Genome Biology* published a study stating that the combination of diesel exhaust and high cholesterol can increase the risk for heart attack and stroke far more than the exposure to either one alone. The study explains how fine particles in air pollution can interact with low-density lipoprotein (LDL, "bad cholesterol") and create a dangerous synergy that results in blood vessel inflammation and hardening of the arteries. One can only imagine what this means for millions of urbanites with stressful jobs and long commutes on congested highways. High cholesterol runs rampant in the United States—feeding a billion-dollar industry that hawks statins, which are cholesterol-lowering drugs, as miracle drugs. An estimated 12 to 15 million American adults of every age and description depend on these drugs daily. They have become among the most popular prescription drugs in America.

Relying on statins, however, isn't a fail-safe solution. They can reinforce unhealthy habits (eating processed foods high in saturated fat, salt, and refined sugars) and serve as a disincentive to create a healthy lifestyle. Moreover, there are hidden risks to statins that don't get publicized nearly as much as their touted benefits. For example, in August 2003, the FDA approved a statin drug called Crestor (rosuvastatin calcium). But because high amounts of it can cause muscle destruction that may lead to kidney damage (and failure), it can be prescribed only in small doses and requires doctors to monitor a patient's muscle enzymes and kidney and liver functions every three months. (For more about toxins and pharmaceutical drugs, see Appendix C.)

A connection has also been found between exposure to cadmium and lead and an increase in cholesterol levels. Animal studies reveal that in the presence of these heavy metals, cholesterol becomes less mobile in the body, resulting in high levels of triglycerides in the blood. This is why paying attention to your heavy metal exposure and doing the detox program targeting heavy metals is important if you have a family history of cardiovascular disease, or if you've already had personal experience with heart trouble in the past.

THE REPRODUCTIVE SYSTEM

Last summer, *Vogue* magazine published its "Age Issue" with a cover story that got a lot of women talking. The story was titled "An Inconceivable Truth: The Link Between Infertility and the Environment." And it brought a host of facts and truths to light that many devoted readers of the magazine probably had never considered.

We have long blamed women's infertility on timing matters—a woman who waited too long to have children or who cannot point to a medical condition and is thus somehow personally at fault. But now that more women are talking about their struggles with pregnancy and the topic is less taboo, we are seeing some incredible statistics that are grabbing the attention of public health officials, politicians, and fertility experts.

At least 10 percent of all couples in the United States cannot conceive a child, and this percentage appears to be increasing. Also on the rise are tubal pregnancies and in vitro fertilization clinics reporting abnormal embryos being produced by young, "healthy" women in their twenties. In fact, women in their twenties are more likely than ever to have trouble getting pregnant. According to the National Center for Health Statistics, a 42 percent jump in fertility problems was reported between 1982 and 1995.

Women in the prime of their childbearing years aren't the only ones having trouble with fertility. Studies are now pouring out of various institutions showing connections between exposure to toxins and male infertility as well. Sperm rates have fallen in much of the industrialized, Western world. They've declined more so in places where pesticides are prominent, and male infertility reports are mounting like never before. Environmental exposure to heavy metals also has been the target of a few studies. One such study, published in a 2003 issue of *Human Reproduction,* reported that lead may be behind up to a fifth of unexplained male infertility cases. Researchers found evidence that even low-level lead exposure from household contaminants (e.g., lead-based paints, piping, plumbing fixtures, and contaminated soil) may damage sperm and contribute to male infertility.

Epidemiologist and biostatistician Shanna Swan, Ph.D., of the University of Rochester School of Medicine has spent the past twenty years studying environmental reproductive risks. In 2003, while at the University of Missouri at Columbia, she reported that men in rural Missouri had a 42 percent lower sperm count than those who lived in cities like Minneapolis and New York. In another study, this one conducted by researchers for the North Shore–Long Island Jewish Health System headquartered in Great Neck, New York, 40 percent of men with unexplained infertility tested high for lead in both blood and semen—higher than what is acceptable even for someone who is exposed to lead at work.

The percentage of infertility cases that have no clear, underlying reason currently stands at 10 percent. And now that the data are emerging to show links between increases in infertility and the rise in ubiquitous chemicals, people are beginning to take note and doctors are now looking for clues in food, water, and the home. The very things that make up the fabric of our lives may be largely responsible for our progressively more defunct health and "fecundity," which is how scientists refer to the ability to procreate.

Without a doubt, researchers will continue to explore the effects of pollution on pregnant mothers, fetuses, and adults in general. In the past several years, numerous studies performed on female agricultural workers exposed to copious amounts of pesticides have shown a remarkably increased rate of spontaneous abortions and stillbirths.

We know now that the developing fetus is exceptionally vulnerable to the effects of toxic metals, chemicals, and pesticides to which the mother is exposed. As it turns out, many heavy metals, including lead and mercury, can cross the placental barrier and do significant damage—much more so than the same dose taken in by the mother. Prenatal and infant mercury exposure, for example, can cause mental retardation, cerebral palsy, deafness, and blindness. Even in low doses, mercury may affect a child's overall development, delaying walking and talking, shortening attention span, and causing learning disabilities.

Lead exposure presents a unique situation. Because lead is similar to calcium in structure, it takes the place of calcium during the development of the nervous system in a growing fetus. The results can be devastating, causing serious disorders that are echoed in later behavioral and learning problems. The mother is also affected by this lead-calcium interaction, which can cause high blood pressure and a reduced production of red blood cells that are critical for carrying oxygen throughout the body and to the fetus. The good news is that studies show that dietary nutrients can decrease the transfer of toxins to the fetus during pregnancy, making a stronger case for pregnant moms to pay greater attention to their diets. A mom-to-be would do well to heed the diet recommendations set forth in the Detox Diet with its focus on nutrient-rich foods that are whole and unprocessed. The changes you will make as you complete the RENEW program and adopt a healthier lifestyle will put the power in your hands for fulfilling a life of health and passing that health on to your children.

THE ENDOCRINE SYSTEM

One word encapsulates what the endocrine system is about: hormones. Physiologically, hormones control much of what you feel—moody, tired, hungry, hot, or cold. Women who are reading this know exactly what I'm talking about, and for that matter I am sure the men reading this know, too. The endocrine system regulates development, growth, reproduction, and behavior through an intricate system of hormones. Hormones are your body's messengers that get produced in one part of the body, such as the thyroid, adrenal or pituitary gland, pass into the bloodstream, and go to distant organs and tissues, where they act to modify structures and functions. They essentially act like traffic signs and signals—telling your body what to do and when so it can run smoothly and efficiently. They are part of your reproductive system as well as part of your urinary, respiratory, cardiovascular, nervous, muscular, skeletal, immune, and digestive systems.

And when hormones run amok, you will notice it. They can go wild naturally during stressful periods or as a result of your age and condition (think puberty, pregnancy, menopause, et cetera), or they can become imbalanced under the influence of toxins that mess with the body's innate hormonal machinery, much like a drunk driver who can't operate a car.

First, toxins tend to accumulate in endocrine glands and in fatty tissues (e.g., breasts). Second, when the liver is loaded down with too many toxins, it can begin to clear them less efficiently from the body, especially excess estrogen. And because hormones have such a command over so many functions in the body, a disruption can result in myriad problems: metabolic imbalances, thyroid disorders, infertility, fibroids in both the breast and the uterus, cysts, cancer, insulin resistance or sensitivity, diabetes, endometriosis, premenstrual syndrome, hypoglycemia, prostate conditions, insatiable cravings, and so on. The list continues, and these problems are actually precursors to other problems, including unexplained weight gain or loss, chronic pain, irritability and mood instability, hair loss, fatigue, a loss of libido, and a general sense that something isn't right. You feel tired and weak, unable to participate in life to its fullest. In a nutshell: you feel gloomy and slightly depressed.

The most pernicious toxins that continue to accumulate in our environment and that wreak havoc on our endocrine system are the so-called hormonal disrupters, such as the estrogenic pesticides that mimic the female hormone estrogen, and antiandrogens that antagonize the male hormones, including testosterone. Pesticides that are similar in chemical structure to our natural estrogen and impersonate estrogen's effects in the human body can have disastrous consequences. The largest area of estrogen receptor sites is located in the breast tissue. Although they are similar in structure to estrogen, these compounds, once in the breast tissue, can contribute to cellular changes and mutation of breast tissue cells. What does that mean? It means breast cancer.

Antiandrogens are capable of preventing or inhibiting the biologic effects of androgens on normally responsive tissues in the body. They usually work by blocking the appropriate receptors, competing for binding sites on the cell's surface, and thus obstructing the androgens' pathway. In the presence of antiandrogens, which are found in commonly used fungicides for agriculture, a developing fetus will generate gene mutations that then change the genital organs. If the fetus is male, he could be born with both male and female characteristics; a female may look nearly normal but have undescended testes. People with this disorder, called androgen insensitivity syndrome, may struggle for years with their sexual identity. Many opt for surgery to help physically clarify whether they are male or female.

Thyroid disorders can also initiate a bevy of health problems. At the center of the thyroid's activity is thyroid stimulating hormone, which can be disrupted by fungicides and other chemicals such as perchlorate, which we saw earlier finds its way into our food and water supplies. This commonly found chemical greatly increases a woman's risk of hypothyroidism and can disrupt the thyroid's ability to absorb iodine.

Diabetes belongs under the umbrella of the endocrine system because it occurs when the body can no longer produce or use normally the pancreatic hormone insulin. As you know, cases of diabetes continue to increase dramatically not only across the United States but also globally. While it's the sixth leading cause of death, it just may be the most preventable and reversible disease of the bunch—particularly Type 2, or adult-onset diabetes, which often occurs with lack of exercise, poor diet, and obesity. (The link between diabetes and obesity and these two diseases' impact around the world is why we are hearing the term "globesity" now.) Type 2 diabetes occurs when the body loses its ability to keep blood sugar levels under control. Insulin is supposed to encourage cells to take sugar out of the blood. When diabetes is present, the body becomes insulin resistant— unable to respond to insulin's efforts to reduce blood sugar. The major health consequences of diabetes include heart disease, stroke, blindness, kidney failure, pregnancy complications, lower-extremity amputations, and death.

What really gets me is the number of people projected to have diabetes in the future: One in three Americans born in the year 2000 will develop adult-onset diabetes. As the United States population gains weight, including record numbers of children, the tremendously increased incidence of this debilitating disease is causing many doctors and leaders to worry that the word *disaster* rather than just *epidemic* is looming ahead. Already diabetes now kills more people than AIDS; and the total number of people with diabetes is expected to double globally, from 171 million in 2000 to 366 million in 2030.

In my last book, *The Fiber35 Diet: Nature's Weight Loss Secret*, I went into detail about how and why a fiber-rich diet can help prevent, manage, or even reverse diabetes. But while many already realize that diet and exercise are two of the biggest factors when it comes to the risk for diabetes, both of which are largely under an individual's control, you may not know that toxins can also have an impact. Several studies worldwide have examined the relationship between environmental influences and diabetes, turning up astounding findings. These discoveries have led experts to conclude that we cannot blame diet and a sedentary lifestyle alone for diabetes. But it's important to note that all three potential causes can combine to have a profound impact on the individual risk. As you progress through the RENEW program, you will find that it addresses all three areas. It's nearly impossible to clean up the toxins in your personal world without cleaning up your diet and boosting your activity level. All three habits—nourishing your body with superfoods, revving up your metabolism through exercise, and doing what you can to limit your exposure to toxins—must work in synch. They will create a magical alchemy for you that paves your path to a healthy, happy body.

THE MUSCULOSKELETAL SYSTEM

We may be living in an increasingly aging society, but the numbers of people who suffer from muscle and joint pain, fibromyalgia, and arthritis is remarkable, especially when you consider the numbers of young people dealing with health issues previously thought to afflict only the elderly.

Arthritis, you'll recall, is the leading cause of physical disability in the United States, and despite what you might think, arthritis is not just an "old person's" problem. The prevalence of arthritis today is enormous, and its causes are more complex than age and genetics. Arthritis comprises more than 100 different disease and conditions. The most common are osteoarthritis, rheumatoid arthritis, fibromyalgia, and gout. It has been estimated that as many as 70 million Americans—or about one in three— have some form of arthritis or joint pain. Here's a surprising fact: Adults sixty-five years of age or older have the highest risk of arthritis, but two-thirds of all people with arthritis *are younger than sixty-five.*

Due in part to the permeability of the synovial membrane, which is the layer of cells and connective tissue that encloses a freely movable joint and secretes the lubricating synovial fluid, many organisms can infect the joints, such as bacteria, viruses, infections from other areas of the body, chemicals, cellular waste, and even digestive toxins. Once inside the synovial fluid, these foreign invaders can cause joint pain, inflammation, and stiffness, otherwise known as arthritis. Some people also experience a toxic reaction to specific foods like bell peppers, tomatoes, and eggplant, triggering arthritic pain.

Accumulation of heavy metals and toxins within the body tissues also has been linked to numerous pain conditions. Although the exact cause of fibromyalgia is still unknown, toxicity of the body from chemicals, pesticides, air pollution, and toxic elements are believed to be a big causative factor. Many people, through detoxification programs, have a reduction or complete eradication of fibromyalgia.

THE NERVOUS SYSTEM

Any chemical, pesticide, heavy metal, solvent, and so on that causes adverse effects on the nervous system is considered a neurotoxicant. To date there are 1,179 chemicals currently registered and used in the United States that are listed as known or suspected neurotoxicants, and you come into contact with them every day.

The effects toxins can have on our nervous system is sweeping, similar to the all-encompassing effect they can have on the endocrine system. In addition to our nerves and spinal column, at the top of the nervous system is the organ that controls so much of our life: the brain. Anything that disrupts the brain's health and capacity to function normally should be a cause of alarm.

First, a note about fat. If there's one kind of "body fat" that's extremely healthy, it's the kind that comprises our nervous system. Yes, you read that right: about two-thirds of your brain is composed of fats. And the protective sheath that covers communicating neurons is composed largely of fat—70 percent fat, to be exact—and the rest is protein. When you digest the fat in your food, it's broken down into fatty acid molecules of various lengths. Your brain then uses these for raw materials to assemble the special types of fat it incorporates into its cell membranes. It especially likes healthy fats such as omega-3s and -6s. This is why it's very important that we get essential fatty acids from our diets from foods such as fish, avocado, almonds, walnuts, flaxseed, and olives. They are essential because your body can't manufacture them on its own. This gives a whole new meaning to the term "brain food," which is how many people refer to fish, because it often contains high-quality fat.

But because fat is a building block to the nervous system, this makes it vulnerable to fat-soluble toxins. Heavy elements such as elemental mercury vapor and many pesticides are "lipophilic," or fat-loving (they dissolve in fat much as two different oils can merge seamlessly together). So these fat-loving toxins, once in the blood, will eventually migrate to a fatty area of the body—to fat cells, to bone marrow, and to every corner of the nervous system, including the brain. While it's true that the blood-brain barrier is designed to act like a gatekeeper, protecting the brain from toxins trying to enter, many toxins sneak by due to their highly lipophilic nature. Some can quite easily attach themselves to a carrier protein, as if they were disguising themselves and hitching a ride, which then passes this barrier and lands in the vulnerable brain.

Once toxins are in the brain, they may have difficulty passing back out due to the blood-brain barrier. They can accumulate inside the brain tissue and eventually disrupt normal brain function, most notably causing damage to the cells, disrupting normal brain chemicals and neurotransmitters, and damaging the myelin sheaths protecting the nerves in the brain. This in turn can cause such disease processes and conditions as depression, anxiety, learning disorders, autism, ADHD, multiple sclerosis, and brain diseases such as Alzheimer's and Parkinson's. Poor memory, "brain fog," and unexplained numbness can also be the results of toxins impinging on an otherwise healthy nervous system.

Autism and Vaccines?

This is a hotly debated topic today. Autism, which afflicts a record 1 in 150 children, involves the destruction of the myelin sheath surrounding the nerve fibers in the brain. The myelin sheath develops from early childhood and is a prominent weak point for toxic damage, especially mercury. It's believed to result from disruption of normal neurobiologic mechanisms primarily in the prenatal period and is widely recognized to have a strong genetic component.

The number of children reported with autism, from mild to severe cases, has increased dramatically especially during the last ten years, but scientists disagree on how much of this increase represents actual incidence and how much may be due to increased awareness and diagnosis. Nonetheless there continues to be lively debate about environmental roots of autism, which may have nothing to do with genetics. When California researchers, for example, studied the association between autism and environmental pollution in the San Francisco Bay area, they discovered a potential connection between ambient metal concentrations, and possibly chlorinated solvents, and an increased risk for autism.

A lot of controversy has also emerged concerning the mercury preservative called thimerosol used in vaccines, as some believe it can cause autism. There is no doubt that certain forms of mercury, including the ethyl mercury used in thimerosol, passes through the blood-brain barrier and can accumulate in and possibly damage the brain. We still don't know yet the origins of autism but it's curious to see a rise in autism alongside a rise in environmental toxins. Many doctors are no longer using vaccines containing thimerosol, but you must be specific when requesting them for your children.

THE IMMUNE SYSTEM

The human immune system is a vast and complex area of continued study. The variables of immune parameters from one individual to the next makes the study of environmental and occupational exposure on human immune function somewhat difficult. That said, there are some definitive links being made between exposure to environmental factors and the effects of those factors on the immune system. Four hundred twenty-six chemicals known or suspected to poison the immune system are currently registered in the United States alone.

The immune system is our main line of defense against disease. But when the immune system cracks, it leaves us at the mercy of invaders and sometimes even its own internal demise through the bewildering progression of autoimmune disorders such as lupus, rheumatoid arthritis, and MS. Studies have shown that mice exposed to relevant doses (i.e., doses equivalent to what a human might encounter) of the solvent trichloroethylene, used in adhesives, paint removers, and spot removers, and found in many water sources from dumping of the chemical, developed lupuslike symptoms and autoimmune hepatitis.

Autoimmunity confuses many people, but it's simply an inappropriate immune response to the body's own tissue that can eventually lead to tissue damage and dysfunction. The immune system can become dysfunctional in two ways—overstimulation and suppression. Synthetic chemicals can do both, depending on the specific chemical at hand. An overworked (overstimulated) immune system, for instance, may prompt the system to turn on itself, activating allergies or autoimmune diseases. Conversely, a suppressed immune system is an open invitation for viruses, parasites, and bacteria that can cause minor problems such as colds, flus, and respiratory infections, or a major disease like cancer. Researchers have found that many pesticides interfere with most white blood cell and antibody formation, decreasing the body's resistance to infections. Household pesticides have come under fire following a study that showed a strong association between the use of professional pest control services at any time while a child is between the ages of one and three and a significantly increased risk of childhood leukemia. Numerous studies of exposure to the chemical benzene, one of the world's major commodity chemicals, have demonstrated a radically elevated risk of leukemia.

Given the important role our immune systems play in keeping us healthy and disease free, clearly, when we weaken our immune systems, we weaken our ability to deal with our "body burdens" All of the steps in RENEW address the immune system either directly or indirectly, keeping it as strong and fully equipped as possible.

AN END TO TOXIC STRESS

Let's recap the big picture to bring this conversation to a conclusion. As we've covered, the barrage of toxins to which we're exposed today, virtually everywhere on the planet, but especially in industrialized societies, is unprecedented. This excessive exposure means that our livers are under more stress than the livers of our parents and grandparents. Such stress increases our nutritional needs, but, sadly, today's standard diet of refined, enriched, preserved, irradiated, genetically modified, pasteurized, homogenized, hydrogenated, and otherwise processed foods doesn't begin to meet our increased nutritional needs. Today's foods are less nutritious than their counterparts of yesteryear, owing largely to methods employed by modern agribusiness to increase agricultural yield and shelf life—at the expense of nutrient content and consumer health.

The combined stresses of nutrient depletion and toxicity lead to liver stress, dysfunction, and ultimately disease. The daily toll that is taken on our livers by undernutrition (often coupled with overeating) and toxic overload is not immediately apparent. It is possible for a person whose liver function is compromised by as much as 70 percent to have no symptoms, nor any clinical sign of liver impairment. While people with hepatitis or cirrhosis have obvious liver disease, it is not widely recognized that those with chronic diseases such as cancer, diabetes, arthritis, and osteoporosis generally have poor liver function as well. Remember, liver dysfunction can give rise to virtually any disorder, for it adversely affects the digestive, immune, hormonal, circulatory, and nervous systems in a variety of ways.

When the liver is toxic and congested, fats are not metabolized properly. This can lead to an obstruction of blood vessels, high blood pressure, heart attacks, and stroke. As fat builds up in the liver and other organs, metabolism (conversion of food to energy) slows down, resulting in weight gain (especially in the belly) and unsightly cellulite deposits.

Because a toxic liver is not filtering properly, it is unable to rid the bloodstream of undigested food particles that have arrived there via a leaky gut, giving rise to an autoimmune response. (Leaky gut syndrome is a condition in which one's intestinal lining becomes semi-permeable; spaces develop between the cells of the gut wall—permitting bacteria, toxins, and food to leak through.) Thus, a person with a toxic liver will be prone to allergies (the net result of this process), slowly becoming allergic to virtually everything if steps aren't taken to detoxify the liver. Blood sugar problems (both hypoglycemia and adult-onset diabetes) are common in those with a fatty liver; so are depression, brain fog, indigestion, constipation, bloating, recurrent infections, chronic fatigue, fibromyalgia, and more.

Since the liver is our central line of defense against toxins, when it is overworked, an extra load is placed upon our other organs of detoxification. That extra load is passed from one organ system to another until either detoxification occurs, enabling the body to regain balance, or degeneration sets in. Many years ago, the late master herbalist Stuart Wheelwright dubbed this domino effect the "toxic stress cycle."

As medical researchers learn more about toxins, a growing consensus focuses on the central role toxins play in damaging our health. They take a toll from the time you are in your mother's womb until you take your last breath. What's more, they may even harm you before you are conceived.

It's remarkable to think that exposure of an embryo to environmental toxins can create new inherited traits, but scientific research has shown this to be the case. In other words, if your great-grandparents were exposed to toxins in utero, the traits that have been handed down to you may have been damaged by toxins. And if you are pregnant, toxins that you (and your growing baby) are exposed to may cause damage in your great-grandchildren. This makes the call to action much more imperative. The steps you take today to clean up your environment and your body may ultimately have an impact on the future health of your loved ones. You will also be doing your part in effecting change on a global scale. I applaud you for taking action. You will bring your body—and your world—into a more balanced, healthy state.

Chapter 10 Summary

*

- Toxins not only overwhelm the liver; they also affect nearly every bodily system, including

  - digestive
  - respiratory
  - cardiovascular
  - reproductive
  - endocrine
  - musculoskeletal
  - nervous
  - immune

- Illness and disease related to these systems can be rooted in toxin overload.

- Ending the toxic stress cycle that opens the door to illness starts with proper detoxification.

- A commitment to routinely addressing your body's detoxifying needs through a program like RENEW can help lower your risks for age-related disease and award you a lifetime of vibrant health.

*

CHAPTER 11

THE RENEW RECIPES

❧

Your detoxification program with the herbal supplements will be greatly enhanced if you clean up your diet and follow the guidelines outlined in Chapter 6. In a nutshell, this means focusing on organic foods, lean proteins, and fiber-rich produce. Embrace all-natural options, including wild-caught fish, and do your best to avoid processed foods that contain refined sugars, preservatives, additives, and unhealthy fats. Also don't forget to severely cut down on or forgo sugary beverages, caffeine, and alcohol. You have plenty of options for staying hydrated using natural ingredients.

❧

In this chapter you'll find some of my favorite recipes attuned to the recommendations of the diet so you can learn how to put these concepts together into a doable eating plan. I'll also be giving you my juicing and shake recipes that will further aid your detoxification. They are great complements to meals or as standalone snacks. Remember, you do not have to follow a strict diet protocol while you are on the herbal cleansing regimens. I only include these recipes (and the menu ideas found on pages 158-159) as a way of teaching you how to prepare healthy, delectable meals without the fuss. Choosing to eat well does not have to entail extra work or time in the kitchen. Once you get used to this way of eating, which is truly delicious, it can become a way of life that's deeply satisfying. Continuing on a path to better, more vibrant health will be relatively effortless.

Feel free to play with these recipes and find your own personal versions based on your likes and dislikes. Unless otherwise noted, recipes are for one serving, but you can choose to double or triple any of these if you want to make more for storage or your family.

BREAKFAST

Nutty Rice Porridge

½ cup	long-grain brown rice
1 cup	almond milk
¼ teaspoon	ground nutmeg
¼ cup	chopped walnuts
2 tablespoons	ground flaxseed
½	Fuji apple, chopped (Fuji apples are best for their texture and sweet taste, but you can choose another type of apple)

Place the rice, milk, and nutmeg in a medium saucepan. Bring to a boil, stirring frequently.

Cover pan and reduce heat to low. Simmer for approximately 45 minutes. Top with chopped nuts, ground flaxseed, and apple.

Eggless Veggie Omelet

You can make this with any vegetables you like.

16 ounces	firm, water-packed tofu, rinsed
1 tablespoon	extra virgin olive oil
1 ½ tablespoons	Bragg Liquid Aminos or soy or tamari sauce
¼ teaspoon	dry mustard
1 clove	garlic, minced
1 small	shallot or onion, diced
½ cup	sliced crimini mushrooms
½ cup	green, red, or yellow peppers
	Sea salt and fresh ground pepper to taste

Using paper towels, blot as much moisture from the tofu as you can.

Heat a skillet over medium-high heat. Add the olive oil so that the bottom of the skillet is coated.

Break the tofu into bite-size pieces and add them to the hot skillet, stirring occasionally so that the tofu browns evenly, about 5 to 10 minutes.

Sprinkle in the Bragg Liquid Aminos, garlic, dry mustard, sea salt, and pepper. Toss evenly to season. Add vegetables and toss until tender.

LUNCH

Grilled Salmon and Endive Salad

(Serves 4)

1 cup	radicchio
2 cups	curly endive, endive, or romaine lettuce
1 cup	fresh pineapple slices
1 cup	fresh mango slices
½ cup	red onion, sliced
2	leek bulbs, sliced (peel off and discard outer leaves; wash leeks thoroughly)
4	wild salmon fillets (4 to 6 ounces each)
	Sea salt and ground pepper to taste

Preheat grill to high heat. Make a tray out of heavy-duty foil large enough for the salmon fillet (fold a long piece in half and fold up all four sides, with the dull side up). Spray the entire inside of the foil tray liberally with organic, olive-oil cooking spray. Drizzle olive oil on top of the fillet with dash of salt and fresh ground pepper. Place foil tray on hot grill and cook (covered) for 10 minutes per 1 inch thickness of the fish. Turning is not necessary. Salmon is done when it turns a light pink color throughout and feels firm when pressed gently with the back of a fork. Remove and cover to keep warm, clean off grill, and prepare vegetables.

Place vegetables and fruit on grill or you can use a sauté pan. Heat on both sides for about 2 minutes, just enough to make them a little limp. Place all the ingredients on a platter or large bowl, drizzle with dressing (recipe follows), and top with the grilled salmon.

Honey Lime Dressing

In a small bowl, combine the juice of 1 lime, 1 teaspoon honey, chopped mint to taste, sea salt and pepper to taste, and 1 garlic clove, minced. Add ½ cup extra virgin olive oil in a slow stream, whisking until blended. This is a good basic dressing for almost any salad. Store in a glass container in the refrigerator with a tight-fitting lid for up to 1 week.

Grilled Tempeh with Mixed Greens

(Serves 4)

8 ounces	organic tempeh (of any type), cut crosswise into 1⁄4-inch slices
1 tablespoon	extra virgin olive oil
¼ teaspoon	sea salt
8 cups	mixed salad greens (organic if possible)
½ cup	thinly sliced yellow bell pepper (about 1⁄2 medium)
1	leek bulb, thoroughly washed and thinly sliced
1 pint	small cherry or grape tomatoes

Lightly brush both sides of tempeh slices with olive oil and sprinkle with sea salt. Heat on a grill or in a grill pan over medium–high heat approximately 4 to 6 minutes per side, until grill marks appear and the tempeh begins to brown. Remove from heat.

Cut grilled tempeh strips into bite–size pieces. Set aside.

Combine mixed greens, yellow pepper, leek, and tomatoes in a large bowl. Drizzle the dressing (recipe follows) over greens and top with the tempeh.

Spicy Tamari Orange Dressing

2 tablespoons	tamari
1 tablespoon	honey
	Juice of 1 orange
½ cup	extra virgin olive oil
	sea salt to taste
1 dash	ground red pepper
1 clove	garlic, minced

In a blender, place tamari, honey, orange juice, olive oil, sea salt, fresh ground pepper, and garlic clove, minced. Blend until smooth.

DINNER

Dover Sole Roll-ups

1 ½ pounds	sole fillets (approximately 6 fillets; you want pieces about 1/4 inch thick and 2 to 3 inches wide)
2 to 3	fennel bulbs, thoroughly washed and sliced very thin
1 large	red pepper, sliced lengthwise in strips
1 tablespoon	fennel seeds, crushed
	Sea salt and pepper to taste
¼ cup	sliced almonds

Place sole on a chopping block. Layer the sole with sliced fennel, and a few strips of red pepper. Sprinkle each piece with the crushed fennel, sea salt, and pepper. Roll from end to end and use a toothpick to secure. Place in a buttered shallow glass baking dish and cover with foil.

Bake at 425°F until fish is opaque but moist-looking in the center, about 12 to 16 minutes.

Meanwhile, toast the almonds by heating them in a skillet, stirring occasionally, until brown. Set aside and prepare the sauce (recipe follows).

White Wine Shallot Sauce

In a 10- to 12-inch pan over medium heat, stir together 2 tablespoons extra virgin olive oil and 2 tablespoons minced shallot until golden brown, about 3 minutes. Add ¾ cup white wine or chicken stock. Boil on high heat, stirring occasionally, until reduced to ¼ cup, 5 to 7 minutes.

When the fish is done, remove the foil, drizzle with the sauce, and sprinkle toasted almonds on top.

Roasted Blackened Salmon

This recipe is wonderful served with steamed asparagus (see below).

4 (4-ounce)	wild salmon fillets
1 teaspoon	blackened seasonings (store-bought varieties of blackened seasoning mixes are fine)
2 teaspoons	tamari
2 tablespoons	chopped fresh cilantro (or to taste)
1 medium	shallot, finely chopped

Preheat oven to 450°F.

Lay salmon on a baking sheet or broiler pan. Brush with the tamari and sprinkle with the blackened seasonings. Bake for 10 to 11 minutes per 1 inch thickness of fish. It should be just cooked through. Salmon will be light pink in color and firm when pressed with the back of a fork. Remove, and immediately sprinkle with cilantro and shallots. Let stand for a few minutes and serve.

Steamed Mediterranean Asparagus

1 bunch	asparagus, woody stems (approximately 25 medium spears or 50 petite spears)
1 tablespoon	extra virgin olive oil
	juice of ½ fresh lemon
	sea salt and pepper to taste

In a sauté pan on medium heat, lay asparagus all in the same direction. Add a small amount of water and cover. Steam until tender, about 3 minutes. Remove from heat and sprinkle with sea salt and pepper, olive oil, and lemon juice.

Almond Brown Rice with Orange

This is delicious with any fish!

2 ¼ cups	chicken stock (you can also use vegetable stock)
1 cup	brown rice
	sea salt to taste
½ cup	sliced almonds
	zest of one orange
	juice of one orange
1 tablespoon	extra virgin olive oil

Bring the chicken stock to a boil and add brown rice. Bring back to a boil, then reduce heat to medium-low. Simmer while covered for about 40 minutes, or until rice fluffs with a fork. Season with sea salt and add the almonds, orange zest, juice of the orange, and olive oil. Toss until thoroughly blended and serve.

The Detox Broth

I make this Detox Broth in a large quantity and then store it in a glass container in the refrigerator with a tight-fitting lid. It will keep for up to 5 days. Full of nourishing nutrients that aid in the body's natural detoxification, this broth is also a great way to stay hydrated (it counts toward your daily water intake). Drink either with meals or in between.

12 cups	filtered water
8 cups	chopped and mixed organic vegetables, such as burdock root, red beet, sweet potatoes, carrots, onions, celery, any sea vegetables, daikon, turnip, parsnips, shiitake mushrooms, and garlic (whole bulb)
	Fresh herbs and spices, such as cilantro, ginger, cayenne pepper, lemon grass, parsley, oregano, and fennel

Add water, herbs, and veggies to a large stockpot and bring to a boil. Reduce heat and simmer for a few hours.

Strain in a sieve or fine-mesh filter bag, often referred to as a nut milk bag.

Drink warm 2 to 3 cups a day.

J U I C E S

Juicers can be found in many large retail and specialty stores for kitchen and house wares. They run the gamut in terms of price, power, and functionality. I recommend doing some homework prior to purchasing a good juicer if you don't already have one. Some, for example, are better at juicing whole fruits and vegetables than others. Some can be extremely versatile, suitable for making pasta, baby food, and nut butters.

The following recipes are for one serving, but each can yield different amounts depending on the size and quality of your fruits and vegetables. Because juicing extracts so much concentrated juice, it's important to use organic produce whenever possible—especially if skins and rinds are involved as they can harbor chemicals from sprayed pesticides.

Keep your fruits and vegetables in the refrigerator if you like your juice cold, and be sure to wash them thoroughly before placing them in the juicer. It helps to have a staging area on your countertop with all your ingredients placed on one side of the juicer ready to go. Most juicers are dishwasher-friendly, but try to clean and wash out your juicer at least by hand soon after you are done preparing the beverage. If you use your juicer frequently, it may be better to wash by hand so it's ready to go the next time; or you can choose to double or triple the recipes below and store leftovers in the refrigerator. They will keep up to three days.

A note on ginger: This is a strong-flavored root so you get to choose how much "a small section" means to you. One to three inches of this root will yield approximately one-quarter to one whole teaspoon of ginger juice. If you want more (or less) of this refreshing flavor in your drink, simply adjust the amount of ginger in your recipe to meet your preferences.

Citrus Cocktail

¼	lemon with peel
½	grapefruit (peeled)
2	oranges (peeled)
Small section	fresh ginger with peel

Basic Blend

¼	head red or green cabbage
3	celery stalks

Red Detox

2 to 3	carrots
½	beet
1 leaf	swiss chard, kale, or collard

Fresh Garden Tonic

4	carrots
1	apple
2	celery stalks
½ handful	wheatgrass
2 sprigs	parsley
½	beet
1 leaf	swiss chard, kale, or collard
Small section	fresh ginger with peel
Pinch	cayenne pepper

Sweet Body Cleanse

2 to 3	carrots
½	beet
½	cucumber

Cucumber Refresher (for healthy hair, skin, and nails)

1	cucumber
3	kale leaves or any dark green such as mustard greens, broccoli, or collard
4	carrots
¼	green pepper

Pineapple Cooler

4 to 5	pineapple rings
½ cup	sparkling water

Tropical Spritzer

1	mango
Small section	fresh ginger with peel
½	lime with peel
	Add sparkling water to finish

HIGH-FIBER
SHAKES AND DRINKS

The following shakes pack a powerful punch of good nutrition. Each offers a delicious blend of high-quality protein, fiber, and the natural juice from fruit to keep you energized and satisfied. As with all the recipes, these are great to have whether you're actively detoxing with the herbal supplements or not. They take minutes to prepare and can be snacks or simply complement a snack or meal. (I love them in the afternoon when that late-day lull hits and I begin to crave something sweet and filling.)

You'll find protein-fiber shake mixes at most grocery stores, especially those that specialize in organic or natural foods. Look for a brand that contains whey protein and feel free to play with different flavors if, for example, you want to try a chocolate-flavored shake over vanilla. If you're having trouble finding mixes with high fiber, it's okay to go with a high-quality protein powder and then add your own fiber. You can do this easily by throwing in a scoop (or two) of flaxseed meal or a fiber supplement in powder form. If you prefer icy shakes over thinner ones, just add more ice or choose frozen fruit over fresh. You may also choose to mix in water instead of milk where indicated.

Use the following recipes as guidelines, and see if later on you can create your own tasty blends based on personal references for fruit and protein mix flavors.

Peach Shake

2 scoops	protein-fiber vanilla shake mix
4 ounces	almond milk
4 ounces	filtered water
½ cup	organic peaches, diced fresh or frozen

Combine and mix in a blender.

Cherry-Vanilla Shake

2 scoops	protein-fiber vanilla shake mix
4 ounces	soy milk
4 ounces	ice
½ cup	pitted black cherries, fresh or frozen

Combine and mix in a blender.

Pea Protein/Multinutrient Drink

1 scoop	pea protein/multinutrient
6 ounces	fresh apple juice
6 ounces	filtered water, almond milk, soy, or rice milk
1 tablespoon	flax oil

Combine and mix in a blender.

APPENDIX A

Please Pass the Pesticide

Pesticides have long been used in commercial agriculture to protect crops from damage by insects. Unfortunately, residues of those pesticides remain on the harvested crops and ultimately end up in our bodies. The National Cancer Institute has repeatedly found that farmers have higher than average risks for several types of cancer affecting the blood (leukemia), brain, and stomach. They also have been shown to suffer from higher than average rates of depression or suicide.

Agricultural toxins like pesticides, herbicides, and fungicides, as well as synthetic chemical additives (including hormones and antibiotics) that change our foods at the source—on the farm in soils and animals—continue to be a major concern, so much so that organic foods are quickly becoming mainstream across America in most regular grocery stores now that we are demanding higher-quality products. I just hope that federal regulators continue to keep the standards high when it comes to the term organic. Now that corporate food giants such as Dole, General Mills, Kraft, and ConAgra have gotten into the "organic" game, they have, as part of an industry-wide group, lobbied hard to change the rules about what it means to be "organic." If they win at getting synthetic chemicals like ripening agents and thickeners added to the list of allowable ingredients, or even genetic engineering to pass muster, then "organic" will move further and further away from "pure."

In 1996, the two houses of Congress unanimously enacted the Food Quality Protection Act (FQPA). Through this historic action, Congress presented the EPA with the immense challenge of implementing the most comprehensive overhaul in decades of the nation's pesticide and food safety laws. The centerpiece of Congress's challenge was the requirement to review and reassess—within a decade—the tolerances (maximum permitted residues) for all food-use pesticides to ensure they met a new, strict safety standard.

Prior to the FQPA, the laws governing food safety were a bit fuzzy, or at least they allowed for a lot of leeway. The Delaney clause, named after Congressman James Delaney of New York and tacked onto the Federal Food, Drugs, and Cosmetic Act in 1958, said, "the Secretary [of the Food and Drug Administration] shall not approve for use in food any chemical additive *found to induce cancer in man, or, after tests, found to induce cancer in animals.*" Not any. Zero. That may sound like a bold statement to make and a clause difficult to bend, but in fact, plenty of abuses of this clause did occur. There were plenty of loopholes to be found that resulted in lots of known carcinogens ending up in foods.

Thankfully, the FQPA kick-started an overhaul of the system and by the end of 2006, the Pesticide Program had reassessed more than 99 percent of the 9,721 subject tolerances. This entailed an effort that included the detailed review of tens of thousands of toxicology, chemistry, and environmental studies as well as the application of new risk assessment methods and policies. Good news: this ten-year effort, based on sound science and broad public participation, resulted in the strictest protective standards for pesticide regulation for all Americans, especially infants and children. More than 4,300 individual pesticide registrations were canceled because they were deemed unsafe (a good thing!).

But there are still more than 1,300 chemicals registered as pesticides in the U.S. These chemicals are formulated into thousands of pesticide products that are used agriculturally and available in the marketplace for home usage. In both 2000 and 2001, the total amount of pesticide used in the U.S. was approximately 5 billion pounds. We must remain vigilant about pesticide exposure in our surroundings and lives in general.

Just recently, in the summer of 2007, research revealed a correlation between higher rates of autism and mothers exposed to the organochlorine pesticides endosulfan and dicofol.

The study found that the closer an expectant mother lived to places where these pesticides were used the greater the risk that her children would develop autism spectrum disorder. The timing of exposure was also found to be critical, with the exposure during the first trimester of pregnancy—when critical structures are developing in the brain—carrying the greatest risk of autism (the chances were 6.1 times greater than for mothers not exposed to these chemicals). Researchers noted that the size of the increase in autism risk—a sixfold increase—is much larger than scientists are accustomed to seeing in studies of this kind.

These two commonly applied pesticides are used on cotton, grapes, tomatoes, lettuce, alfalfa, citrus, beans, and other fruit, nut, and vegetable crops. Dicofol, listed as a potential carcinogen, is similar to DDT in its structure, and both are suspected endocrine disruptors. Acutely toxic, endosulfan is up for inclusion in the Rotterdam Convention, an international treaty requiring special import notifications for a list of problematic chemicals, and was recently nominated for global phaseout under the international Stockholm Convention.

Similar stories abound:

- In the fall of 2006, two high school students designed their science fair project around monitoring the air for pesticides by an elementary school. The school was adjacent to fields of Chinese cabbage in an agricultural area in Hastings, Florida. They detected both the insecticides endosulfan and diazinon, as well as the herbicide trifluralin.

- Tired of seeing their children become ill during times of peak pesticide spraying, a group of concerned residents in California tested the air they breathe and their own bodies for the presence of the commonly used, highly toxic pesticide chlorpyrifos. More than 91 percent of the people tested had above average levels of breakdown products of chlorpyrifos in their urine, and most of the women had amounts above the level calculated from EPA data to be safe for pregnant and nursing women. Community members currently are calling for stronger protections from chlorpyrifos and other high-hazard pesticides, including establishing protection zones between residential areas and fields that are sprayed, and notification laws for applicators so that residents can be warned before spraying occurs. They are also asking the EPA and the California State Department of Pesticide Regulation to phase out and eliminate chlorpyrifos for agricultural uses. A phaseout of all domestic uses of chlorpyrifos was completed in 2005—a decision based largely on the health hazards it posed to children—yet chlorpyrifos is still widely used in agriculture, and the threat of exposure remains high for rural residents, including children.

- Lindane may have been banned in fifty-two countries, but it's still used today in the United States and persists in the environment. The EPA no longer allows its use as a pesticide in agriculture, describing it as one of the most toxic, persistent, bioaccumulative pesticides ever registered, yet the FDA continues to allow its use in lice treatment shampoos for *children*. What's ludicrous is that this highly toxic chemical cannot be used on plants and pets anymore, yet we permit it on children's heads (where it can readily be absorbed through the skin). Lindane, the active ingredient in many prescription lice treatments, is a neurotoxic chemical in the same family as DDT. Like DDT, lindane remains in the environment, collects through the food chain, and travels on air and water currents to pollute the farthest reaches of earth. It blocks specific sodium channels, causing overstimulation of the body, and breaks down into several metabolites, one of which is readily stored in body fat. A 2003 study by the CDC determined that 62 percent of Americans have the insecticide in their bodies. Lindane is implicated in causing cancer, fetal toxicity, birth defects, reproductive problems, aplastic anemia (a blood disorder), kidney damage, and endocrine disruption; lindane also is acutely toxic to aquatic life. A higher incidence of breast cancer has been found in areas where lindane is used extensively.

Despite all the health risks and warnings, pesticides continue to be used extensively throughout the world. In the United States alone, more than 18,000 products are licensed for use, and each year more than 2 billion pounds of pesticides are applied to crops, homes, schools, parks, and forests. Such widespread use results in pervasive human exposure. If you were born before 1974, you may have been exposed to dieldrin, a pesticide that was found in 96 percent of all meat and 85 percent of all dairy products tested in the United States. If you were born before 2004, you may have been exposed to diazinon, a toxin poisonous to the nervous system and sprayed on lawns and in gardens before its ban.

There is reason to believe (and hope) that ultimately, the "pest" problem on farms may be solved not through the use of more potent pesticides but through restoration of optimal mineral balance to the soil in which crops are grown. (As an aside, I want to share what Keith S. Delaplane, a professor of entomology at the University of Georgia, says about "pests": "In nature, there are no pests. Humans label as 'pests' any plants or animals that endanger our food supply, health or comfort. To manage these pests, we have 'pesticides.' These are products 'intended for preventing, destroying, repelling, or mitigating any pest [according to the Federal Act].'"

Just as we are coming to recognize the importance of the condition of the body's terrain (internal environment) to health, so too are we becoming increasingly aware that the health of plants is dependent upon the condition of the soil (external terrain) in which they're grown.

Chemical "NPK" fertilizers (composed of nitrogen, phosphorous, and potassium) have been widely used in agriculture for over a century. These fertilizers stimulate plant growth by returning just three minerals to the soil, which normally contains scores of minerals. In this way, the soil is made deficient in those critical trace minerals that are not resupplied. This is similar to the situation we have created by "enriching" refined foods. After the refining process strips the food of dozens of critical nutrients, that food is "enriched" through the addition of just four nutrients (B_1, B_2, niacin, and iron, in a synthetic form). Here again, a situation of imbalance is created, which makes the deficiency worse, rather than correcting it.

NPK fertilizer further affects the soil adversely by acidifying it, which has the net effect of killing off soil microorganisms whose job it is to break up and transmute, or change the nature of minerals for use by the soil. Without these critical microbes, soil minerals become locked up, and the health of the soil declines. Consequently, plants become malnourished, sick, and easy prey for insects. Here we may make another comparison: overacidified soil is like the human body that has become overly acidic as a result of eating a junk food diet. Such a body also becomes prey to "bugs"—in the form of germs. The body that is overly acidic is toxic, for many toxins are of an acidic nature. By continually consuming commercial produce that is grown on nutrient-deficient soil and carries traces of toxic pesticides, we are further adding to the toxic burden carried by our bodies.

Common Effects from Pesticide/Insecticide Exposure

- headache
- nausea
- dizziness
- skin irritation
- coughing
- shortness of breath
- throat/nose/mouth/eye irritation
- metallic taste in mouth
- bad breath
- bizarre or aggressive behavior
- loss of appetite
- muscle weakness
- abdominal pain
- giddiness
- lethargy
- diarrhea
- confusion
- excessive salivation and tearing
- muscle twitching
- pulmonary edema
- seizures
- numbness
- blurred vision
- excessive sweating
- slow heartbeat
- excitability
- disorientation
- nasal bleeding
- slurred speech
- itching
- blood in urine
- tarlike feces

Unfortunately, clinicians on average receive fewer than four hours of training in the important field of occupational and environmental health. Although some health workers may be familiar with the management of acute pesticide poisoning, chronic effects of pesticide exposure are often overlooked. Acute dermatitis is the second most common occupational disease for all industrial sectors. The rates of dermatitis in the agricultural industry are the highest in any industrial sector.

APPENDIX B

The Cancer Connection

Cancer still holds the number two spot on the list of top killers of adults; it is the number one cause of death in children. At the beginning of the twentieth century, the incidence of cancer was about 1 in 50 in the United States. Today, the risk of an American man developing cancer over his lifetime is currently one in two (leading cancer sites for men are prostate, lungs, and colon and rectum); approximately one in three women will develop cancer over her lifetime (leading sites for women are the breasts, lungs, and colon and rectum). And, like so many other diseases that could be preventable, cancer and toxins have a long, correlative history in scientific literature.

The relationship between toxins and cancer are well documented—for many types of cancer, including leukemias and lymphomas, and for virtually all types of toxins. In fact, in response to the public's request for information regarding the relationship between environmental factors and the development of cancer, the National Cancer Institute (NCI) and the National Institute of Environmental Health Sciences (NIEHS), two departments of the National Institutes of Health, created a booklet titled *Cancer and the Environment*. It contains information about environmental substances either known or suspected to cause cancer. As a result of their research they found that as many as two-thirds of *all* cancer cases are linked to environmental causes.

Cancer is responsible for nearly a quarter of all deaths (heart disease claims a little more than that at 27.2 percent, and the next runners-up fall way behind these leading two killers). Here is just a small sampling of facts that illustrate the mind-boggling growth in cancer rates:

- Sometimes called the "silent epidemic," over the last several decades incidences of **non-Hodgkin's lymphoma (NHL)** have been increasing by 3 to 4 percent *per year* throughout most of the world. In some studies annual increases are as high as 4.2 to 8 percent. These reported increases are corrected for known viral causes of NHL, such as human immunodeficiency virus (HIV), and therefore largely exclude AIDS-related lymphomas. Such annual increases translate to about a 250 percent increase in the last fifty years.

- The age-adjusted incidence of primary **tumors of the central nervous system** (CNS) (particularly astrocytomas, including the rapidly progressive glioblastoma multiforme as well as the benign meningiomas) appears to have increased by 50 to 100 percent over the past several decades, with the greatest increase ocurring among the elderly.

- The United States has recently experienced increased incidence of and mortality from **renal cancers**. According to Surveillance, Epidemiology and End Results (SEER), a national cancer monitoring program, the last twenty-five years have witnessed dramatic increases in disease and death from kidney cancer among black and white Americans of both sexes. During the last twenty years, all white men saw increased incidence at 3.1 percent *per year*; white women at 3.9 percent; and African-American men and women the steepest rate at 3.9 percent and 4.3 percent. Such increases over a twenty-year period cannot be explained by early detection, especially given that screening tests are not routinely employed.

- **Testicular cancer** is another malignancy rising in occurrence for the last several decades in virtually all developed nations. The nation's oldest ongoing statewide tumor registry finds a mean annual increase in testicular cancer incidence of more than 5.5 percent over the last sixty years. New studies are showing that a mother's exposure to pollutants may contribute to testicular cancer in her sons years later.

- Age-adjusted incidence of **breast cancer** in industrialized countries has increased 1 to 2 percent *per year* for several decades, both before and after the introduction of mammography.

- **Prostate cancer** is up nearly 290 percent in the last fifty years.

- **Thyroid cancer** is up 258 percent.

- Cases of **skin melanomas** are up almost 700 percent in the last fifty years.

- **Lung cancer** is currently the most common cause of cancer death in women, with the death rate more than two times what it was twenty-five years ago.

In the last fifty years, incidence of age-adjusted cancer increased roughly 85 percent in the United States. Because this figure is adjusted for age, people living longer has nothing to do with this increase. The most affected part of the population is children, who represent the fastest-growing sector of people with unprecedented high rates of cancer. Every year approximately eight thousand children under age fifteen are diagnosed with a malignant disease, most frequently leukemia and brain tumors. Environmental exposure such as to ionizing radiation, hormones, and antineoplastic agents are accepted to be contributors to these diseases. At this writing it is estimated that about 1.4 million new cases of cancer will have been diagnosed in 2007. Cancers of the prostate and breast will be the most frequently diagnosed cancers in men and women, respectively, followed by lung and colorectal cancers both in men and in women. Overall, the most common cancers—skin, lungs, breasts, kidneys, colorectal and prostate—are organs of excretion. It's possible that toxin accumulation for purpose of excretion may be a clue as to the connection between toxins and excretory organs.

APPENDIX C

Medical and Dental Toxins

We tend to make a distinction between "good" drugs (legal ones) and "bad" drugs (illegal ones), but the fact of the matter is that all drugs, even prescription and over-the-counter drugs, are toxic to some degree. While a medicine may effectively relieve an unpleasant symptom, the price paid in terms of potential side effects (both felt and unfelt) may be great. This fact is dramatically reflected in a lengthy and well-documented report compiled by medical doctors and researchers with the Nutrition Institute of America and presented a detailed analysis of medical literature and government health statistics released in 2003. In their paper, the team reports that the number of people who died in 2001 as a result of "iatrogenic" conditions (those brought on inadvertently by either medical treatment or diagnostic procedures) was greater than that of the number of people who died in that same year of either heart disease or cancer, the number one and two leading causes of death in the United States respectively. The numbers were as follows:

Deaths from cancer	553,251
Deaths from heart disease	699,697
Deaths from medical treatment	783,936

The report further states that "over 2.2 million people are injured every year by prescription drugs alone, and over 20 million unnecessary prescriptions for antibiotics are prescribed annually for viral infections." Overuse of antibiotics has led to the development of antibiotic-resistant organisms and has the net effect of reducing a patient's immune response because beneficial intestinal bacteria are eliminated.

Then came another report in 2007 from researchers at the Institute for Safe Medication Practices in Huntingdon Valley, Pennsylvania, stating that deaths or injuries related to drug treatments more than doubled between 1998 and 2005 in the United States, with painkillers and immune-system boosters accounting for most. Their findings, which were published in the *Archives of Internal Medicine*, were based on "serious adverse drug events" (those that cause death, birth defects or disability, resulted in hospitalization, or were life-threatening) as reported to the U.S. Food and Drug Administration.

Even drugs that are generally recognized as safe, such as aspirin, can cause serious side effects. Aspirin belongs to a class of drugs known as nonsteroidal anti-inflammatory drugs (NSAIDs), which irritate the stomach lining, can cause ulcers and lead to leaky gut syndrome, thus permitting potentially damaging nonnutrient substances to gain access to the bloodstream. In fact, NSAIDs are one of the leading causes of stomach ulcers, and their misuse leads to more than 100,000 hospitalizations and more than 16,000 deaths each year in the United States. Acetaminophen, for example, which many people wrongly assume is among the safest drugs of all, has been proven to cause liver damage when taken in excess. Steroids (such as cortisone and prednisone), also used to combat inflammation, may lead to deterioration of the intestinal lining. Researchers have also found that people share a concern today for side effects associated with over-the-counter pain relievers, but at the same time those same people admit to taking more than the recommended dose.

If you are like most people, you throw away the original box and any paper that comes with your over-the-counter medicine. Very few people save leaflets or packaging with important warning information. But even conscientious people who read the fine print may not get the crucial information they need. That's because many nonprescription drug labels are woefully inadequate.

For example, if you compare the official prescribing information for prescription Motrin with the over-the-counter variety (Motrin IB) label, you find that many warnings and precautions are left out. Doctors read about such side effects as edema, blurred vision, nausea, heartburn, diarrhea, gastric ulcer with bleeding and/or perforation, dizziness, nervousness, rash, and tinnitus ("ringing in the ears"). On the OTC Motrin IB box, side effects are not specifically listed. There is a mention that "ibuprofen may cause stomach bleeding," and that people should "stop use and ask a doctor if stomach pain or upset gets worse or lasts." But research has shown that most people don't want to bother their doctors with questions about nonprescription drugs. Warnings about drug interactions are also grossly incomplete. This means you take on serious risks when you take OTCs blindly; OTCs can be just as hazardous to your health as prescription medications.

Many medications, whether prescribed or over-the-counter, adversely affect the body's detoxification organs, chief of which is the liver. Renowned hepatologist and liver disease specialist Melissa Palmer, M.D., tells us that there are more than a thousand drugs and chemicals that can cause injury to the liver, thus compromising the body's detoxification capabilities. In fact, some drugs are so injurious to the liver that doctors must weigh the pros against the cons when deciding whether or not to pursue a certain treatment. Sometimes the drug can be more problematic than the disease or infection itself. Current drugs, for instance, used to help prevent the development of tuberculosis in someone who has tested positive for exposure to this bacteria, are extremely taxing on the liver. Even an otherwise healthy young person may have to go through the drug treatment process with his or her liver function in constant check.

You may have noticed the deluge of advertisements from drug companies in the media in the past several years. Direct-to-consumer ads is a new trend and one that is predicted to strengthen; in 1997 drug companies spent about $1 billion on direct-to-consumer ads, but by 2004 that number had increased to more than $4 billion. Drug companies rely so much on profit generated from drugs, especially new ones attached to active patents, that they've begun persuasive marketing campaigns targeting consumers directly. In doing so, many times they will angle an ad to make you think you need this pill or that potion to live a healthier, longer life (as in "Ask your doctor if X is right for you.") Little do pharmaceutical companies care about the repercussions of having so many people hooked on drugs that may have side effects and consequences, as well as heighten your risk for more health problems (that then require more drugs). At the same time, we are likely to see the FDA continue to loosen its grip on which drugs should be prescription-only and which ones will be available over the counter (already, seven hundred more medicines are accessible today over the counter than what was available thirty years ago).

Coupled with this trend is a concurrent rise in the number of people who are self-diagnosing and self-medicating, which sets the stage for millions of people to overtreat themselves and suffer untold penalties with regard to their health. Unfortunately, because medicine and its delivery is largely a reactive industry driven by huge insurance companies that wait until you get sick before allowing coverage to kick in, we've grown accustomed to being reactive patients. We wait until we get sick to seek solutions to our health problems.

As this book reiterates throughout, the natural approach to health and healing is attuned with the body, working with it rather than against it. This was the philosophy of many traditional remedies that have now been lost or replaced. In the RENEW program you will come to understand how the body is equipped to heal itself through uniquely designed detoxification methods. In combination with proper nutrients, exercise, and other habits, you can help determine the direction your body takes—to optimum or downgraded health.

Many drugs can inhibit each other's clearance from the body, causing toxic, elevated amounts of each to be stored in cells, notably in the liver and kidneys. Moreover, in today's world where people do a lot of self-medicating with over-the-counter drugs (more of which continue to spill onto the market as drug companies lose patents and the FDA loosens its rules on what should be prescribed or not), the risk for unwittingly overburdening your body is much bigger.

Add to that the fact we'd like to think anything over-the-counter is "safe" and we've got ourselves a recipe for disaster. As people mix drugs coming in from various doctors (a heart medication from their cardiologist, a sleeping aid from their internist, and a painkiller from their rheumatologist), the toxic blend can be dicey for a liver not designed for the load. Granted, it can likely endure a certain load of toxins to some degree, especially during a small period of exposure. But it's the long-term strain you put on your liver that can mean the difference between health and chronic illness. Or life and death.

It's common knowledge that any kind of drug "overdose" can have damaging, even fatal, effects. But it's not common knowledge exactly what "drugs" can cause damage to the liver and/or kidneys that can build up over time and go from minor to serious and life-threatening. Everyday drugs used to help alleviate pain or an unwanted symptom like a runny nose from allergies can and do harm your body's natural ability to detoxify as well as operate an effective digestion and elimination process. In addition, there can be numerous intertwining effects happening with the taking of several drugs. You take drug A to relieve symptom B, but drug A triggers effect C, for which you now pop drug D, and so on and so forth.

Let me give you another example. Constipation is a common side effect of many medications. It can result from ingestion of antidepressants, pain medications, diuretics, antibiotics, and antacids that contain aluminum. Antacids, however, can further aggravate the very symptoms they're taken to alleviate (i.e., heartburn, indigestion). They also inhibit phase I detoxification in the liver (discussed in Chapter 4) and can cause damage to this organ. Constipation is but one of many symptoms that can result from antibiotics, which destroy both good and bad bacteria in the digestive tract. Antibiotic use can result in overgrowth of yeast and fungus with the attendant problems. Use of tetracycline, a commonly prescribed antibiotic, can cause development of fatty deposits in the liver, which is the hallmark of an unhealthy liver on the road to cirrhosis. Erythromycin, another commonly prescribed antibiotic, can cause cholestasis, or diminished bile flow.

So it can be a vicious cycle of injury and reinjury. What's more, the demand your liver endures as you continue to consume more and more toxins in the form of drugs can become so overwhelming that it begins to shut down. And once that happens, a cascade of physical ailments that entails other organs and systems will likely follow.

Following are common "drugs" that your liver must process. The more toxins your liver meets, the more it has to work, and the more stress it has to bear (i.e., the bigger your body burden gets). All this can translate to significant wear and tear that ultimately compromise your body's ability to effectively process toxins and support a healthy system on all fronts—from digestion and elimination to your heart, lungs, and other vital organs.

- alcohol
- antihistamines
- benzodiazepines (Halcion, Centrax, Librium, Valium, etc.)
- birth control pills
- caffeine
- laxatives
- marijuana
- NSAIDs (nonsteroidal anti-inflammatory drugs, including aspirin, ibuprofen, and naproxen sodium)
- sleeping pills
- steroids (cortisone, prednisone, anti-inflammatories)
- tobacco

Don't panic. As I said at the end of the test you took in Chapter 1, don't begin to agonize if you currently use or have used one or more of these drugs on the list. My RENEW program will help you minimize your need for these drugs in your life—even if you must continue using a particular prescription drug and even if you choose to drink coffee and alcohol. In all likelihood you will not need to resort to many of these drugs once you renew your body. And you will learn how to make slight shifts in your lifestyle to accommodate the drugs you may still choose to use, while also continuing on your path to a healthier, more vibrant you.

As previously noted, dental materials and procedures also make a significant contribution to the body's toxic load, thereby creating disease conditions. An increasing number of progressive physicians are beginning to believe that a good portion of chronic disease has its roots in dental toxicity. While the best-known toxic dental material in use today is the controversial "silver" amalgam, which is over half mercury, many other potentially damaging metals (especially nickel and palladium) and nonmetallic restorative materials are also in widespread use in dentistry today. Progressive dentists are continually seeking and finding safer ways to practice dentistry by refining standard techniques and by testing materials for biocompatibility—i.e., making sure that the materials are safe for the individual patient.

RESOURCE DIRECTORY

Note: The following is a listing of recommended sources, Web sites, and organizations. It is a comprehensive guide of trusted resources, but it is by no means complete. It would be impossible to list every resource available to you, which is why I invite you to explore options in your local area. Don't forget to also go to www.detoxstrategy.com for updated information and help in finding the best products to support your detoxification program and overall health.

Toxin Testing

Doctor's Data, Inc.
www.doctorsdata.com
800-323-2784

Lab Testing Direct
www.labtestingdirect.com
877-223-0102

Lab Safe
www.labsafe.com
888-333-LABS
(888-333-5227)

Functional Testing

Genova Diagnostics
(endocrinology, gastrointestinal, immunology, nutritional, metabolic testing)
63 Zillicoa Street
Asheville, NC 28801
828-253-0621
www.gdx.net

Detoxification Centers

Hippocrates Health Institute
1443 Palmdale Ct.
West Palm Beach, Florida 33411
561-471-8876
www.hippocratesinst.com

We Care Spa
18000 Long Canyon Rd.
Desert Hot Springs, CA
800-888-2523
www.wecarespa.com

Gerson Institute
1572 Second Ave.
San Diego, CA 92101
Phone: 619-685-5353 /
888-443-7766 (U.S. only)
800-838-2256 (toll-free, U.S. and Canada)
Fax: 619-685-5363

Renew Life
1007 N. Macdill Ave.
Tampa, Florida 33607-5126
813-871-3200
rclinic2@tampabay.rr.com

Optimum Health Institute
San Diego, CA
800-993-4325
www.optimumhealth.org

Environmental Health Center
Dallas, TX
William Rea, M.D.
214-368-4132
www.ehcd.com

MercOut International, Ltd.
2583 E. Sunrise Blvd.
Ft. Lauderdale, FL 33304
www.mercout.com

Professional Organizations

Centers for Medicare & Medicaid Services
7500 Security Blvd.
Baltimore, MD 21244
www.cms.hhs.gov

Centers for Disease Control and Prevention (CDC)
1600 Clifton Rd., N.E.
Atlanta, GA 30333
404-639-3311/
800-CDC-INFO or 800-232-4636
Public inquiries: 404-639-3534
www.cdc.gov/about

Commonweal
PO Box 316
Bolinas, CA 94924
415-868-0970
commonweal@commonweal.org

Environmental Working Group
Headquarters
1436 U St., N.W., Suite 100
Washington, DC 20009
202-667-6982

California Office
1904 Franklin St., Suite 703
Oakland, CA 94612
510-444-0973
www.ewg.org
www.ewg.org/sites/humantoxome/index.php

The Institute for Functional Medicine
4411 Pt. Fosdick Dr. NW, Suite 305
PO Box 1697
Gig Harbor, WA 98335
800-228-0622
www.functionalmedicine.org

Healthy Child Healthy World
12300 Wilshire Blvd., Suite 320
Los Angeles, CA 90025
Phone: 310-820-2030
Fax: 310-820-2070
www.healthychild.org

International Association for Colon Hydrotherapy
PO Box 461285
San Antonio, TX 78246-1285
Phone: 210-366-2888
Fax: 210-366-2999
www.i-act.org

U.S. Environmental Protection Agency
Ariel Rios Building
1200 Pennsylvania Ave., N.W.
Washington, DC 20460
www.epa.gov

Natural Resources Defense Council
40 West 20th St.
New York, NY 10011
Phone: 212-727-2700
Fax: 212-727-1773
www.nrdc.org

National Institutes of Health (NIH)
9000 Rockville Pike
Bethesda, Maryland 20892
www.nih.gov

Organisation for Economic Cooperation and Development
2, rue André Pascal
F-75775 Paris, Cedex 16, France
Main switchboard, tel.: +33-1.45.24.82.00
Fax: +33-1.45.24.85.00
www.oecd.org

Pesticide Action Network North America
49 Powell St., Suite 500
San Francisco, CA 94102
Phone: 415-981-1771
Fax: 415-981-1991
www.panna.org

World Health Organization (WHO)
Avenue Appia 20
CH - 1211, Geneva 27, Switzerland
Phone: +41-22 791 2111
Fax: +41-22 791 3111
www.who.int/en/

U. S. Food and Drug Administration (FDA)
5600 Fishers Lane
Rockville MD 20857-0001
888-INFO-FDA (888-463-6332)
www.fda.gov/

Helpful Web sites

Second Look
For a bibliography of scientific literature on fluoride, go to
www.slweb.org/bibliography.html

The Agency for Toxic Substances and Disease Registry (ATSDR)
www.atsdr.cdc.gov

Air Now (for air quality index and information)
www.airnow.gov

Chemical Industry Archives, a project by Environmental Working Group
www.chemicalindustryarchives.org

Environmental Health Perspectives
www.ehponline.org

United States National Library of Medicine, Environmental Health and Toxicology
http://sis.nlm.nih.gov/enviro.html

The Right-to-Know Network, which provides free access to numerous databases and resources on the environment
www.rtknet.org/rtkdata.php

Skin Deep, a cosmetic safety database by Environmental Working Group
www.cosmeticsdatabase.com/

The Campaign for Safe Cosmetics
www.safecosmetics.org

Oceans Alive, for list of safe seafood choices
www.oceansalive.org

PAN (Pesticide Action Network) Pesticides Database, for current toxicity and regulatory information for pesticides
www.pesticideinfo.org/Index.html

Natural Resources Defense Council
www.nrdc.org

National Agricultural Statistics Service (NASS), Agricultural Chemical Use Database
www.pestmanagement.info/nass/app_usage.cfm

United States Geological Survey's Pesticide National Synthesis Project
http://ca.water.usgs.gov/pnsp

United States Geological Survey
www.usgs.gov/

Supplies

Air Purifiers

www.air-purifiers-america.com

www.ultra-pureair.com

www.airpurifiers.com/

Water Filtration Systems

www.omni-water-filters.com
1-406-889-5288

www.heartspring.net

www.consumerreports.com

Mail Order Organic Foods

Diamond Organics
1-888-Organic (1-888-674-2642)
www.diamondorganics.com

Papa's Organic
PO Box 7344
Van Nuys, CA 91409
Phone: 818-974-0109
818-890-2497
Fax: 866-shop-papas
www.papasorganic.com

Blackwing, Inc.
17618 W. Edwards Rd.
Antioch, IL 60002
Phone: 847-838-4888
Fax: 847-838-4899
Help line: 800-326-7874
www.blackwing.com

Natural Home Products

Hästens Natural Bedding
Nya Hamnvägen 7
731 23 Köping
Phone: +46(0)221-274 00
www.hastens.com

EcoPlanet—EcoChoices
PO Box 1491
Glendora, CA 91740
Phone: 626-969-3707
www.ecochoices.com/

Gaiam, Inc.
360 Interlocken Blvd., Suite 300
Broomfield, CO 80021
Phone: 877-989-6321
www.gaiam.com

American Pride Paints
Southern Diversified Products, LLC
2714 Hardy St.
Hattiesburg, MS 39401
Customer service: 888-714-9422
www.americanpridepaint.com

Healthy Hues Paints
Healthy Home
2894 22nd Ave. North
St. Petersburg, Florida 33713
800-583-9523
www.Healthyhome.com

Seventh Generation, Inc.
60 Lake St.
Burlington, VT 05401-5218
Phone: 802-658-3773
800-456-1191 (toll-free)
Fax: 802-658-1771
www.seventhgeneration.com

Mrs. Meyers Clean Day
www.mrsmeyers.com

Ecover
800-449-4925
www.ecover.com/us/en/wheretobuy/

Supplement and Natural Product Companies

ReNew Life Formulas, Inc.
198 Palm Harbor Blvd. South
Palm Harbor, FL 34683
800-830-4778
Renewlife.com

Pure Encapsulations
490 Boston Post Rd.
Sudbury, MA 01776
800-753-2277
Purecaps.com

Source Naturals
23 Janis Way
Scotts Valley, CA 95066
800-815-2333 (toll-free)
sourcenaturals.com

Natural Body Care Product Companies

Pangea Organics
Boulder, CO 80301
877-679-5854
www.pangeaorganics.com

MyChelle Dermaceuticals LLC
Box 70
Frisco, CO 80443
800-447-2076
www.mychelleusa.com

Aubrey Organics
4419 N. Manhattan Ave.
Tampa, FL 33614
Phone: 800-282-7394 (toll-free)
Fax: 813-876-8166
www.aubrey-organics.com

NOTES

Introduction: A Time to RENEW
1. To access bulletins, reports, statistics, publications, and data gathered by the World Health Organization, go to www.who.org. Similarly, you can access a wealth of statistical data, general information, and forecasts about diseases as they relate specifically to Americans at the Centers for Disease Control and Prevention Web site at www.cdc.gov.

Chapter 1. How Toxic Are You? Take the Test
1. For more information about the Human Toxome Project and its findings, please go to www.ewg.org/sites/humantoxome/ (or www.bodyburden.org). The project is a collaboration between the Environmental Working Group (www.ewg.org) and Commonweal (www.commonweal.org). The following is the summary of the project's findings:

Study 1: Industrial Chemicals and Pesticides in Adults
- What was tested: In blood and urine: 214 industrial compounds, pollutants, and other chemicals
- Who was tested: 9 adult volunteers from 5 states
- Results: Laboratory tests uncovered 171 pollutants in the blood and urine of each volunteer, including an average of 56 carcinogens in each person.

Study 2: Flame Retardants in Breast Milk
- What was tested: In breast milk: brominated flame retardants used in computers, televisions, and foam furniture
- Who was tested: 20 first-time mothers nationwide
- Results: In the first nationwide test for chemical flame retardants in the breast milk of American mothers, researchers found unexpectedly high levels in every woman tested. Further, milk from several of the mothers had among the highest levels of these chemicals detected worldwide thus far. The breast milk of women tested contained 35 of 44 industrial compounds, pollutants, and other chemicals, including those linked to reproductive and fertility problems, brain and nervous system toxicity, birth defects and developmental delays, and gastrointestinal (including liver) issues.

Study 3: Industrial Chemicals and Pesticides in Adults
- What was tested: In blood and urine: 413 chemicals, including a diverse range of pesticides, flame retardants, and stain- and grease-proof coatings
- Who was tested: A select group of women
- Results: The blood and urine of participants in this study contained 329 of 413 industrial compounds, pollutants, and other chemicals tested, including chemicals linked to brain and nervous system toxicity, cancer, infertility, gastrointestinal problems, immune system responses, and birth defects and developmental delays.

Study 4: Industrial Chemicals and Pesticides in Umbilical Cord Blood
- What was tested: In blood: 413 chemicals, including pesticides, flame retardants, and stain- and grease-proof coatings
- Who was tested: 10 newborn babies, born in U.S. hospitals from August to September 2004
- Results: The cord blood of the participants in the group contained 287 of 413 industrial compounds, pollutants, and other chemicals tested, including chemicals linked to brain and nervous system toxicity, cancer, immune system responses, gastrointestinal problems, and birth defects and developmental delays.

Study 5: Teflon and Mercury in Blood

- What was tested: In blood: Disparate toxins, mercury from tainted fish, and Teflon-like chemicals from consumer products

- Who was tested: 8 volunteers, including teens and adults

- Results: Tests conducted in this study uncovered two extremes in human blood pollution: mercury (an industrial pollutant that accumulates in seafood such as tuna) and Teflon pollution, which has only recently come under intense scrutiny by public health officials. The blood of the participants contained 9 of 14 industrial compounds, pollutants, and other chemicals tested, including chemicals linked to reproductive and fertility problems, cancer, immune system responses, kidney and renal problems, and birth defects and developmental delays.

Study 6: Consumer Product Chemicals

- What was tested: In blood and urine: 70 consumer product chemicals, including plasticizers, flame retardants, and stain-proof coatings

- Who was tested: women and men ages 17 to 71, including 4 mothers and their daughters

- Results: Tests revealed 56 common consumer product chemicals, including plastic softeners, flame retardants, and stain repellents. The blood and urine in each participant from the mother-daughter group contained 56 of 70 industrial compounds, pollutants, and other chemicals tested, including chemicals linked to reproductive and fertility problems, brain and nervous system toxicity, immune system responses, cancer, gastrointestinal problems, birth defects and developmental delays, and hormonal activity.

Study 7: Chemicals in Mother and Two Children

- What was tested: In blood and urine: 304 industrial compounds, pesticides, and chemicals released from plastics

- Who was tested: A mother and two children

- Results: The blood and urine of each participant in this group contained 181 of 304 industrial compounds, pollutants, and other chemicals tested, including chemicals linked to birth defects and developmental delays, cancer, brain and nervous system toxicity, hormonal activity, and immune system responses.

2. Chemical Industry Archives, also run by the Environmental Working Group, hosts a site to help people distinguish between fact and fiction (for example, it's a fact that people vary enormously in their reaction to toxic substances). I invite you to visit www.chemicalindustryarchives.org/factfiction/ to learn more.

3. The average body burden in America is 700 synthetic chemicals from food, water, and air. You can search the Human Toxome database for a chemical's report by browsing chemical classes, exposure routes, health effects, or names at www.bodyburden.org.

4. Numerous studies have demonstrated fetal exposure to toxins. In a revealing study published in the journal *Neurotoxicology* in 2002, researchers identified high levels of eight different insecticides (including DDT, diazinon, lindane, malathion, and chlordane) and three heavy metals (lead, cadmium, and mercury) in the first bowel movements of 426 infants from the Philippines. Further findings revealed that ten of the newborn children had an average of 200 contaminants in their stool, and 209 of the total pollutants found had never before been detected in cord blood. Refer to the following study: E. M. Ostrea et al., "Prevalence of Fetal Exposure to Environmental Toxins as Determined by Meconium Analysis," *Neurotoxicology* (2002) vol. 23, no. 3, pp. 329–39).

According to toxins expert Dr. Doris J. Rapp, unborn babies float nine months in chemicals in the uterus. The same dangerous chemicals, including pesticides, can be found in bowel movements and mother's milk. You can read more about her findings in *Our Toxic World* (Buffalo, New York: Environmental Medical Research Foundation, 2004) or by going to www.drrapp.com.

Also see *Detoxify or Die* by Sherry A. Rogers, M.D. (Sarasota, Florida: Sand Key Company, Inc., 2002).

5. The effects toxins can have on our bodies as we age is tremendous—especially as we gain more fat and lose muscle mass. The more fat we carry, the more toxins we're likely to bear as well. And as our muscle cells shrink, they can release stored toxins, which then can do further damage as they move in the bloodstream.

Dr. Leonard Smith notes that the eyes, in particular, can offer a unique view into toxic metal accumulation. The eyes are, after all, said to be the window to the soul. Age-related macular degeneration (AMD) is the leading cause of visual acuity and blindness after age sixty-five. The eye uses many minerals including zinc, copper, and iron for normal function. But these can be replaced by lead, cadmium, mercury. Much like counterfeit money, these toxic minerals interrupt enzyme pathways and affect mitochondrial function, both essential in maintaining healthy detoxification pathways. So in clinical medicine the eyes provide a window for observing the connections between toxic metal accumulation in the eye, leading to cellular dysfunction and inflammation that result in AMD.

Chapter 2. The Perils of Pollutants and the Power of Detoxification

1. The Toxics Release Inventory is a publicly available database owned by the Environmental Protection Agency and contains information on toxic chemical releases and other waste management activities reported annually by certain covered industry groups as well as federal facilities. You can access this database at www.epa.gov/tri/. The Ecological Rights Foundation also offers a public information site at www.ecorights.org/. Of interest is its "Toxins in Our Environment" and "Toxic Consumer Products" pages (accessed September 15, 2007).

2. The Toxic Substances Control Act (TSCA) of 1976 was enacted by Congress to give EPA the ability to track the 75,000 industrial chemicals currently produced or imported into the United States. You can read more about this act as well as other environmental laws on the EPA's Web site. Specifically, go to www.epa.gov/region5/defs/html/tsca.htm, where you can download the full text of the Act.

3. For more details on individual diagnostic tests that can help determine, for example, how well your body's detoxification processes are operating, refer to Genova Diagnostics in the Resource Directory and the Textbook of Functional Medicine at www.functionalmedicine.org.

4. Mark Hyman, M.D., *Ultrametabolism: The Simple Plan for Automatic Weight Loss* (New York: Scribner, 2006).

5. In a 1971 study, the University of Nevada's Division of Biochemistry determined that chemical toxins weakened by 20 percent a special coenzyme the body needs to burn fat. In a more recent study done in 2002, researchers concluded that toxins released during weight loss had the capacity to damage the fat-burning mitochondria. The damage was significant enough to lower the body's ability to burn calories and, in effect, fat. For leads to clinical studies on the relationship between toxins and fat, weight loss, and metabolism, please see Pelletier et al., "Associations Between Weight-Loss-Induced Changes in Plasma Organochlorine Concentrations, Serum T3 Concentration, and Resting Metabolic Rate," *Toxicological Sciences* (2002) vol. 67, pp. 46–51; and P. Imbeault et al., "Weight Loss-Induced in Plasma Pollutant Is Associated with Reduced Skeletal Muscle Oxidative Capacity," *American Journal of Physiology—Endocrinology and Metabolism* (2002) vol. 282, no. 3, E574–7.

6. The World Health Organization, www.who.org (accessed August 20, 2007).

7. Randall Fitzgerald, *The Hundred-Year Lie: How Food and Medicine Are Destroying Your Health* (New York: Dutton, 2006).

Chapter 3. Step One: Reduce Exposure to Toxins in Your Environment

1. For more information about the risks related to indoor pollution, see www.indoorpollution.com. As far back as 1987 Susan Gilbert, reporting for *The New York Times*, quoted Dr. John Spengler in her article "Home Remedies": "People get hysterical at the thought of hazardous waste sites. But studies show that your risk of getting cancer from exposure to chemicals in the water, paint stripper and other solvents found in your home is greater than your risk from exposure to the same chemicals in a hazardous waste site. And these findings don't just apply to extremely polluted houses." Published September 27, 1987 (accessed at www.nytimes.com in the Archives on October 5, 2007). Dr. Spengler is a professor of environmental health and human habitation at Harvard University.

2. Jeffrey C. May and Connie L. May, *The Mold Survival Guide for Your Home and for Your Health* (Baltimore: The Johns Hopkins University Press, 2004). Online sites that offer information about mold are: www.mercola.com and www.indoorpollution.com/mold_health_problem.htm (accessed September 22, 2007).

3. The National Institute for Occupational Safety and Health is part of the Centers for Disease Control and Prevention. NIOSH is responsible for conducting research and making recommendations for the prevention of work-related illnesses and injuries. To access its information resources and programs, go to www.cdc.gov/niosh/.

4. In 1997, environmentalists released a report titled the "National Coalition Against the Misuse of Pesticides," documenting widespread contamination and poisoning from the single largest pesticide group—wood preservatives—and launched a campaign to stop their use. To access this information, including fact sheets about wood preservatives, go to www.ncamp.org/ and in particular, www.ncamp.org/poisonpoles/factsheet.html.

5. The debate over soy protein and soy-based products continues, and numerous articles and reports have been published. Mary G. Enig, Ph.D., offers an enlightening overview of the subject in her article "The Soy Controversy" accessible at www.westonaprice.org/soy/soy_controversy.html (accessed October 17, 2007). The article first appeared in *Wise Traditions in Food, Farming and the Healing Arts*, the quarterly magazine of the Weston A. Price Foundation, in the summer of 2001. The Food and Drug Administration has also chimed in and I invite you to check out an article published in its consumer magazine titled "Soy: Health Claims for Soy Protein, Questions About Other Components," written by John Henkel and accessible online at www.fda.gov/Fdac/features/2000/300_soy.html (accessed October 17, 2007).

Chapter 4. The Beauty of Your Body's Natural Detox Methods

1. To read a stunning overview about NASH (nonalcoholic steatohepatitis), and to learn other facts and information about the role of the liver, go to the American Liver Foundation's Web site at www.liverfoundation.org. A fact sheet supporting the claims about NASH is available at www.digestive.niddk.nih.gov/diseases/pubs/nash/, see "Nonalcoholic Steatohepatitis," NIH Publication No. 07-4921, November 2006. Also see *Hepatitis Liver Disease: What You Need to Know* by Melissa Palmer, M.D. (New York: Avery Publishing Group, 2000).

Chapter 5. Step Two: Eliminate Toxins in Your Body

1. Brenda Watson, *Renew Your Life: Improved Digestion and Detoxification* (Clearwater, Florida: Renew Life Press and Information Services, 2002).

2. Brenda Watson, *Essential Cleansing for Perfect Health* (Clearwater, Florida: Renew Life Press and Information Services, 2006).

3. The word *chelation* is derived from the Greek word chelè, meaning claw. Chelation as a medical therapy involves the use of chelating agents to detoxify poisonous metals such as mercury, cadmium, arsenic, and lead by converting them to a chemically inert form that can be excreted mostly through the urine and stool without further interaction with the body.

This therapy involves receiving an intravenous chelating agent such as EDTA (ethylenediaminetetraacetic acid), or oral agents such as DMSA (meso 2,3-dimecaptosuccinic acid) or DMPS (2,3-Dimercapto-1-propanesulfonic acid). These three are among the most popular chelating agents in use today.

Whether given orally, or by rectum (as in children) or through an intravenous catheter, these molecules will bind to toxins such as mercury, cadmium, arsenic, lead and aluminum, as well as to beneficial minerals such as calcium, irom, magnesium, zinc, copper, and selenium and more. Thus, a major part of chelation therapy includes periodic monitoring and replacement of beneficial minerals.

It is now common to give either EDTA or DMPS separately or together and then collect urine for 2–6 hours and send it to a speciality lab for analysis. With a challenge test, the levels of mercury, lead, cadmium, arsenic, and aluminum will be higher in the urine than just a random urine or blood toxic mineral test. This is because the toxins bound to the chelating agent are removed not only from the blood, but also from stored toxins in muscles, bones, fat and organs and are excreted in the urine.

The results of the urine chelation challenge test are commonly used by toxicology practiceners as the gold standard for determing the baseline toxic load and for follow up to access the efficacy of their detoxification therapies.

There are opinions in the medical establishment that challenge tests aren't practical since most everyone has stored toxins and many appear to be asymptomatic. However, there are no levels of stored toxins that are considered normal, and it has been well documented that when the toxin levels are lowered many people get markedly better from many different conditions ranging from cardiac arrhythmias to neurologic symptoms ranging from multiple sclerosis to autism.

In fact, according to the DAN (Defeat Autism Now) paper entitled, "Summary of Biomedical Treatments for Autism," the number one treatment for getting better was chelation with 73 percent improvement. This data was collected from a questionnaire from 25,500 parents. (See ARI Publication #34, February 2007 from www.autism.com.) Children have been treated with either DMSA or DMPS orally or with rectal suppositories with good results. This should be done with close medical supervision.

On the other hand, there are several natural chelators that can be taken safely on a regular basis including: glutathione, glutathione precursors (n-acetyl cysteine, glycine, glutamine, and selenium), undenatured whey protein (high in glutathione precursor L-cysteine), lipoic acid (both a chelator and antioxidant that recharges glutathione), curcumin (active ingredient in curry), milk thistle or silymarin (an herb that prevents depletion of glutathione and may increase levels as well), vitamins A,C,E, B vitamins, and the minerals zinc and selenium. In addition there are many foods that help with optimizing detoxification pathways including: broccoli, cauliflower, garlic, onions, eggs, and most vegetables; legumes and grains that are high-fiber foods; and high-quality probiotics. Consumption of these supplements and foods with about half your body weight in ounces of filtered water daily, along with good elimination, will help to eliminate metal toxins on a daily basis. This will become even more important with aging since the detoxification pathways become less efficient.

4. Brenda Watson, *The Fiber35 Diet: Nature's Weight Loss Secret* (New York: Scribner, 2007).

5. The American Association of Cancer Research states that researchers from the Keck School of Medicine of the University of Southern California in Los Angeles, the University of Hawaii in Honolulu, and the University of Helsinki in Finland have shown that, in Mexican-American women, higher intake of dietary fiber is associated with lower circulating estrogen levels. They found that, as dietary fiber intake increases, levels of estrone and estradiol, two female hormones measured in the blood, drop sharply. Because high estrogen levels have been linked to breast cancer, this finding could prove to be a significant step toward preventing breast cancer.

Chapter 6. Step Three: Nourish Your Cells and Systems
1. Interestingly, the U.S. Senate issued a warning to Americans in 1936, stating, "Most of us today are suffering from certain dangerous diet deficiencies which cannot be remedied until depleted soils from which our food comes are brought into proper mineral balance." A great article discussing this problem, which continues to this day, was written by Nataliya Schetchikova for the *Journal of the American Chiropractic Association*, titled "Nutritional Deficiencies." It was published in June 2001 (accessed online at http://findarticles.com/p/articles/mi_qa3841/is_200106/ai _n8963945, October 10, 2007). Information and studies on nutritional deficiencies can also be found at both the National Institutes of Health (www.nih.gov), and the Centers for Disease Control and Prevention (www.cdc.gov).

Chapter 7. Step Four: Energize Your Body, Mind, and Spirit
1. Anne Underwood, "Exercise Helps Reverse Aging: New Research Shows that Exercise Can Help Reverse the Aging Process at the Cellular Level. Strength Training for the Senior Set," *Newsweek*, May 23, 2007. Accessed online at www.msnbc.com (www.msnbc.msn.com/id/18808971/site/newsweek/) on July 10, 2007.

2. For sleep studies as they relate to weight and health, see K. Spiegel et al., "Leptin Levels Are Dependent on Sleep Duration: Relationships with Sympathovagal Balance, Carbohydrate Regulation, Cortisol, and Thyrotropin," *J Clin Endocrinol Metab* (2004), vol. 89, no.11, pp. 5762–71. Also see S. Taheri et al., "Short Sleep Duration Is Associated with Reduced Leptin, Elevated Ghrelin, and Increased Body Mass Index," *PLoS Med* (2004), vol. 1, no. 3.

Chapter 9. Toxic Myths and the Trail of Chemicals in Our Daily Lives
1. The story about the "polluted" Canadian politicians was reported by Martin Mittelstaedt for the *Globe and Mail* in "Ontario Election: Pollutants in Politics. Chemical Testing Reveals Party Leaders' Toxic Relationship," September 9, 2007, accessed online September 10, 2007, at www.globeandmail.com.

2. Judith Berns, "The Cosmetic Cover-Up" as reported May 5, 2004, in *Health Alert Newsletter* by Dr. James H. Martin.

3. Chemical Industry Archives, a project of Environmental Working Group, "Voluntary Chemical Safety Testing: How Self-Regulation Blocked Independent Studies." Go to www.chemicalindustryarchives.org for more.

4. Chemical Industry Archives, a project of Environmental Working Group, "Fact #1: No Health Tests Are Required by Law to Put a Chemical on the Market." Go to www.chemicalindustryarchives.org for more.

5. For an overview about high production volume chemicals, as well as hazard data and more statistics about chemicals, go to www.epa.gov/HPV/pubs/general/hazchem.htm (accessed October 3, 2007). There you'll find astonishing conclusions:

- The U.S. produces or imports close to 3,000 chemicals (excluding polymers and inorganic chemicals)—more than 1 million pounds per year.
- Most Americans assume that basic toxicity testing is available and that all chemicals in commerce today are safe. A recent EPA study has found that this is not a prudent assumption.
- EPA has reviewed the publicly available data on these chemicals and has learned that most of them may have never been tested to determine how toxic they are to humans or the environment.

- International authorities agree that six basic tests are necessary for a minimum understanding of a chemical's toxicity. These tests, called the Screening Information Data Set (or SIDS), cover acute toxicity, chronic toxicity, developmental and reproductive toxicity, mutagenicity, ecotoxicity, and environmental fate.

  - 93 percent of these 3,000 high production volume chemicals are missing one or more of these basic tests.

  - 43 percent of these chemicals are missing ALL of these tests.

  - Only 7 percent of these chemicals have all six of the most basic screening tests.

Additionally, visit the EPA's "New Chemicals Program" to lean more about the management of the potential risk from chemicals new to the marketplace. The program is mandated by Section 5 of the Toxic Substances Control Act (TSCA).

6. Randall Fitzgerald, *The Hundred-Year Lie: How Food and Medicine Are Destroying Your Health* (New York: Dutton, 2006, pp. 23–24).

7. NIH Publication No. 03-2039, printed August 2003, p. 25, "Cancer and the Environment," by the U.S. Department of Health and Human Services, National Institutes of Health, National Cancer Institute, and National Institute of Environmental Health Services. For more about cancer go to the American Cancer Society's Web site at www.cancer.org.

8. For facts and statistics on leukemia, especially as it relates to toxins, refer to the Leukemia and Lymphoma Society at www.leukemia-lymphoma.org, and specifically, www.leukemia-lymphoma.org/all_page?item_id=9346 (accessed September 30, 2007).

9. T. Woodruff, J. Grillo, and K. Schoendorf, "The Relationship Between Selected Causes of Post-neonatal Infant Mortality and Particulate Air Pollution in the United States," *Environmental Health Perspective*, June 1997, 105(6).

10. Dr. James H. Martin, Health Alert (e-bulletin), April 26, 2004 (information taken, in part, from Carol Simontacchi's book *The Crazy Makers: How the Food Industry Is Destroying Our Brains and Harming Our Children* (New York: Tarcher, 2001).

11. For a multitude of studies, data, resources, and general information about air pollution and toxicants, refer to the Environmental Protection Agency at www.epa.gov.

12. M. Birkhoj et al., "The Combined Antiandrogenic Effects of Five Commonly Used Pesticides," Department of Toxicology and Risk Assessment, Danish Institute for Food and Veterinary Research, *Toxicol Appl Pharmacol* (2004) vol. 201, no. 1, pp. 10–20.

13. D. W. Kolpin, "Pharmaceuticals, Hormones, and Other Organic Wastewater Contaminants in U.S. Streams, 1999–2000: A National Reconnaissance," *Environmental Science & Technology*, vol. 36, no. 6, pp.1202–11.

14. D. R. Oros, "Identification and Evaluation of Previously Unknown Organic Contaminants in the San Francisco Estuary (1999–2001)," RMP Technical Report: SFEI Contribution 75, Oakland, Calif.: San Francisco Estuary Institute. Published in 2002.

15. F. D. Houghton et al., "Estrogenicity of Tissue Extracts from White Bass and Channel Catfish Caught in the Three Rivers of Pittsburgh [abstract]." In: American Association for Cancer Research Annual Meeting: Proceedings, Los Angeles, Calif.: AACR, abstract 3458 (2007).

16. The following sites chronicle the Lejeune case of toxic water, both accessed on August 23, 2007: www.atsdr.cdc.gov/sites/lejeune/faq_water.html and www.cnn.com/2007/US/06/12/toxic.tapwater/index.html.

17. In addition to Eric Schlosser's *Fast Food Nation: The Dark Side of the All-American Meal* (New York: Houghton Mifflin, 2001), other facts and information regarding toxic food and related effects have been reported in the following: Daniel Kadlec, "Chain Reaction," *Time*, June 7, 2004, p. 100; Claudia Wallis, "The Obesity Warriors," *Time*, June 7, 2004, p. 89; and Jennifer Warner, "Food Additives May Affect Kids' Hyperactivity," WebMD Medical News, May 24, 2004, reviewed by Brunilda Nazario, M.D., www.webmd.com.

18. For more about fluoride and drinking water, see Barry Groves's *Fluoride: Drinking Ourselves to Death* (Dublin, Ireland: Newleaf, 2002).

19. Facts and figures about the chemical bisphenol A were reported at the following (all accessed on September 16, 2007): www.ewg.org/reports/bisphenola; www.ewg.org/reports/bpaformula; and http://abcnews.go.com/US/story?id=3450831&page=1.

20. To read the story about lead and other toxins in garden hoses, as reported by investigative reporter Lisa Fletcher from ABC News' Phoenix affiliate, go to http://abcnews.go.com/GMA/Consumer/Story?id=3369894&page=1 (posted July 12, 2007 and accessed on October 10, 2007).

21. A fact sheet supporting the claims about NASH is available at www.digestive.niddk.nih.gov; see "Nonalcoholic Steatohepatitis," NIH Publication No. 07–4921, November 2006.

22. For recalls, reports, and alerts on products, refer to the Consumer Product Safety Commission at www.cpsc.gov.

23. William Randall Kellas, Ph.D., and Andrea Sharon Dworkin, N.D., *Surviving the Toxic Crisis* (Olivenhain, Calif.: Professional Preference, 1996, p.176–77).

24. "Diesel Exhaust + Cholesterol = Cardiovascular Disease," Environment News Service, online article published July 26, 2007 (available at www.ens-newswire.com/ens/jul2007/2007-07-26-09.asp, accessed September 2, 2007). Original study citation: K. W. Gong, "Air-Pollutant Chemicals and Oxidized Lipids Exhibit Genome-Wide Synergistic Effects on Endothelial Cells," *Genome Biology* (2007), vol. 8, no. 7, R149.

Chapter 10. Detoxification and Your Health

1. On Feb. 6, 2003, WebMD.com Medical News reported on male infertility and lead exposure: "Lead Linked to Male Infertility, First Clues That Even Low Lead Levels Harm Sperm," which was based on a new study published in *Human Reproduction*. The article is available at http://men.webmd.com/news/20030206/lead-linked-to-male-infertility (accessed September 25, 2007). Also refer to the following study for more: S. Benoff, A. Jacob, and I. R. Hurley, "Male Infertility and Environmental Exposure to Lead and Cadmium," *Human Reproduction Update* (2000), vol. 6, no. 2, pp. 107–21.

2. American College of Gastroenterology Functional Gastrointestinal Disorders Task Force (2002), "Evidence-Based Position Statement on the Management of Irritable Bowel Syndrome in North America," *American Journal of Gastroenterology*, 97(11, Suppl): S1–S26. Also refer to M. Feldman et al., eds., *Sleisenger and Fordtran's Gastrointestinal and Liver Disease: Pathophyiology / Diagnosis /Management*, 7th ed., vol. 2 (Philadelphia: W. B. Saunders), pp. 1794–1806.

3. "Pulmonary Function after Exposure to the World Trade Center Collapse in the New York City Fire Department," *American Journal of Respiratory and Critical Care Medicine*, vol. 174 (2006), pp. 312–19.

4. For more on the effects of lead on fetal development, see the following studies: D. K. Saxena, B. Lal, and S. V. Chandra, "Effect of Lead on Fetal Development in Rats Fed with 8% Casein Diet," *Bull Environ Contam Toxicol* (1987), vol. 39, no. 4, pp. 641–46. Also see Shenggao Han et al., "Effects of Lead Exposure Before Pregnancy and Dietary Calcium During Pregnancy on Fetal Development and Lead Accumulation," *Environmental Health Perspectives*, June 2000 (available at http://findarticles.com/p/articles/mi_m0CYP/is_6_108/ai _63937872; accessed October 14, 2007).

5. Visit www.scorecard.org for volumes of information and statistics on pollution. There you can get an in-depth pollution report for your county, covering air, water, chemicals, and more.

6. Marla Cone, "Study Links Air Pollutants with Autism," *Los Angeles Times*, June 23, 2006 (available at www.wcfcourier.com/articles/2006/06/23/news/breaking_news/d oc449bb1720713e785199982.txt, accessed October 17, 2007). To download a PDF of the study, go to the California Department of Health Services at www.dhs.ca.gov/director/owh/owh_main/pubs_events/news_articles/well_women/6.2006autism.pdf. Another avenue for information is Googling *autism pollution*, and you'll find references to mercury pollution, environmental pollution, and more.

7. P. E. Bigazzi, "Metals and Kidney Autoimmunity," *Environmental Health Perspectives* (1999), vol. 107(Suppl 5), pp. 753–65.

8. Ma Xiaomei et al., "Critical Windows of Exposure to Household Pesticides and Risk of Childhood Leukemia," *Environmental Health Perspectives* (2002), vol. 110, no. 9, pp. 955–60.

9. Pesticides may increase a woman's risk for diabetes during pregnancy, especially when exposed during the first trimester (which for some mothers means getting exposed when the woman may not even know she is pregnant). When the National Academy of Sciences found evidence of an association between the chemicals used in herbicides during the Vietnam War, such as Agent Orange, and type 2 diabetes, the VA announced it had added diabetes to the list of conditions for which Vietnam veterans are eligible for disability compensation. The culprit in Agent Orange that can trigger insulin resistance, which then leads to diabetes, is dioxin, a contaminant in the herbicide used to kill unwanted plants and to remove leaves from trees that otherwise provided cover for the enemy. Studies have shown that dioxin and dioxinlike compounds (DLCs) can cause a variety of illnesses in laboratory animals. More recent studies

have suggested that the chemical may be related to a number of types of cancer and other disorders. (See abstract for "Toxins and Diabetes Mellitus, an Environmental Connection?" at http://spectrum.diabetesjournals.org/cgi/content/abstract/15/2/109. This study was done by a group of researchers at Clemson University Department of Public Health Sciences in Clemson, South Carolina. It was published in *Diabetes Spectrum*, vol. 15, no. 2, 2002.)

Dioxin, however, is not confined to herbicides. Quite to the contrary, it's been a target of study for scientists linking dioxins in our diet to diabetes, because the major source of dioxin for the general population happens to be our diet. Since dioxin is fat-soluble, it bioaccumulates up the food chain and is mainly found in meat and dairy products, including, in order of greatest concentration, beef, milk, chicken, pork, fish, and eggs. Dioxin is highly persistent in the environment. The most toxic form of dioxin is called TCDD, which does not occur naturally and is not intentionally manufactured by industry (except in small amounts for research purposes). But it may be formed during the chlorine bleaching process at pulp and paper mills and with the production of polyvinyl chloride plastics. It is also formed during chlorination by waste and drinking water treatment plants. Dioxin can occur as a contaminant in the manufacture of certain organic chemicals. The major source of TCDD in the environment, however, is incinerators that burn chlorinated wastes. Experts agree that its ubiquity in food, persistence in the environment, and extreme toxicity justify a public health concern. Studies of exposure to TCDD in animals have shown a wide range of severe effects including cancer, immunotoxicity, developmental and reproductive toxicity, liver toxicity, neurotoxicity, skin disease, and loss of body weight. The most noted health effect in people exposed to large amounts of TCDD is chloracne, a severe skin disease with acnelike lesions that occur mainly on the face and upper body.

Another commonly encountered toxin that researchers are just beginning to understand in terms of its relationship to one's risk for diabetes is arsenic. Arsenic is a naturally occurring element that is widely distributed in various compounds throughout the earth's crust. Pure arsenic is a gray-colored metal, but this form is rarely found in the environment. In the environment, arsenic is transported mainly by water. In the United States, it is present in soil and as such, the main exposure to inorganic arsenic in the general population is through the ingestion of high-arsenic drinking water (arsenic combined with other elements, such as oxygen, chlorine, and sulfur, is referred to as inorganic arsenic. Arsenic in plants and animals combines with carbon and hydrogen to form organic arsenic. Organic forms of arsenic are usually less toxic than inorganic forms).

In the general population, exposure to both inorganic and organic arsenic occurs through medicinal, environmental, and occupational routes. Drugs containing inorganic arsenic have been used in the treatment of leukemia, psoriasis, and chronic bronchial asthma and as a tonic, usually at a dose of several hundred micrograms per day. But, as with dioxin, both forms of arsenic are present in varying amounts in food. And seafoods are the main source of arsenic in the diet. They contain relatively high concentrations of organic arsenic and could supply 52 percent or more of the total daily intake of arsenic. (Also refer to the "Toxins and Diabetes Mellitus: An Environmental Connection?" study for more.)

10. Susan Stockton, *ADD: It Doesn't Add Up! Drug-Free Alternatives for Hyperactivity and Aggression* (Clearwater, Florida: Power of One Publishing, 1997).

11. Susan Stockton, *Beyond Amalgam: The Health Hazard Posed by Jawbone Cavitations,* third ed. (Clearwater, Florida: Power of One Publishing, 2001).

12. Susan Stockton, *The Terrain Is Everything* (Clearwater, Florida: Power of One Publishing, 2000).

13. Susan Stockton, *Dynamic Healing through NeuroCranial Restructuring* (Clearwater, Florida: Power of One Publishing, 1999).

Appendix A. Please Pass the Pesticide

1. For data, statistics, and information about pesticides and human health, PANNA (Pesticide Action Network North America; www.panna.org) is an excellent resource. Of note, refer to "New Study Reveals Higher Rates of Autism When Mothers Are Exposed to Pesticides," reported by Stephenie Hendricks, July 30, 2007.

Also see Nancy Nelson's publication, "The Majority of Cancers Are Linked to the Environment," June 17, 2004. Available at www.nci.nih.gov/newscenter/benchmarks-vol4-issue3/page1 (accessed August 28, 2007).

2. U.S. Environmental Protection Agency Office of Pesticide Programs, 2002.

3. Rose Marie Williams reported on lindane in *Townsend Letter for Doctors and Patients*, October 2006. "Lindane: Banned in 52 Countries—Still Used on Kids in U.S.," is available at http://findarticles.com/p/articles/mi_mOISW/is_279/ai_n16865308 (accessed October 17, 2007).

Appendix B. The Cancer Connection

1. A great starting place for all things cancer-related is the American Cancer Society Web site at www.cancer.org.

Appendix C. Medical and Dental Toxins

1. Gary Null et al., "Death by Medicine," *Life Extension Magazine*. Available at www.lef.org/magazine/mag2004/mar2004_awsi_death_02.htm (accessed October 18, 2007).

2. "Reports of Medication Injuries Have Doubled: Study Shows Painkillers, Immune-System Drugs Account for Most Serious Ills," reported by Reuters on September 10, 2007 (accessed at http://www.msnbc.msn.com/id/20697854/ on September 13, 2007). Original source of study: Thomas J. Moore, Michael R. Cohen, and Curt D. Furberg, "Serious Adverse Drug Events Reported to the Food and Drug Administration, 1998–2005," *Archives of Internal Medicine*, vol. 167, no. 16, September 10, 2007.

3. Melissa Palmer, M.D., *Hepatitis Liver Disease: What You Need to Know* (New York: Avery Publishing Group, 2000, p. 377).

ACKNOWLEDGMENTS

This book, as my others, is a result of the extraordinary efforts of many wonderful people, all of whom I could not have survived the process without. I want to extend my personal gratitude and heartfelt thanks to the following: Bonnie Solow, my literary agent, for her ongoing support that has allowed me to continue sharing my message of health to the rest of the world. All my friends at Free Press, including Dominick V. Anfuso, Maria Bruk Aupérin, Martha K. Levin, Carisa Hays, Suzanne Donahue, Sue Fleming, Eric Fuentecilla, Erich Hobbing, Nancy Inglis, Laura Ferguson, Alexandra Noya, and their outstanding sales force. Kristin Loberg, for her amazing creativity and skills and who without, this book would have just been plain words on a page. Dr. Leonard Smith, a wonderful friend and surgeon, whose knowledge and compassion I continue to revere and hope to someday rival. Brenda Valen, my assistant, for all her research, gathering, hard work, and dedication to this project. Michael Black, Jason Oakman, Nip Rogers and the team at Black Sun Studio for their skills, dedication, and support as always. Sandee Kiser, my sister, and Ashleigh Kiser, my niece, for their continued support and creativity with the recipes. Jerry Adams, Bonnie Cooper, Kyle Krukar, Pamela Sapio, and Paul Pavlovich for their participation in all the elements that must come together in a book. To my children, Travis and Joy, and my son-in-law Chris, thank you for all your love and encouragement.

And my biggest thanks goes to my husband, Stan, without whose continued support and praise this book would not have come to completion. Thank you for believing I can do anything. I love you.

INDEX

ABOUT THE AUTHORS

Brenda Watson, C.N.C., is a *New York Times* bestselling author and one of the foremost authorities in the country on internal cleansing and detoxification. She is dedicated to helping people worldwide achieve healthy digestion and leading them on a path toward natural wellness. She lives in Dunedin, Florida, with her husband and their dogs.

Leonard Smith, M.D., is a prominent general gastrointestinal and vascular surgeon, as well as an expert on nutrition and natural supplementation. Dr. Smith believes educating others is an essential part of his role as a doctor and has always incorporated teaching the basics of healthy digestion to his patients.